AQA Home Economics

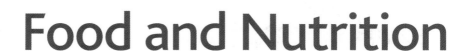

Food and Nutrition

GCSE

Margaret Hague

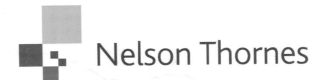

Nelson Thornes

Published in 2009 by:
Nelson Thornes Ltd
Delta Place
27 Bath Road
CHELTENHAM
GL53 7TH
United Kingdom

09 10 11 12 13 / 10 9 8 7 6 5 4 3

A catalogue record for this book is available from the British Library

978 1 4085 0416 1

Illustrations by David Banks and GreenGate Publishing

Page make-up by GreenGate Publishing, Tonbridge, Kent

Printed and bound in China by 1010 Printing International Ltd

Acknowledgements

The author and publisher would also like to thank the following for permission to reproduce material:

Britvic (Fruitshoot); Cadbury; Kellogg's; KP Nuts; Marks & Spencer; Quorn (Marlow Foods Ltd); Somerfield; Waitrose

pp 14, 21, 29 adapted from Bender AE & Bender DA, *Food Tables*, Oxford University Press, 1986; pp 25, 26, 27 adapted from *Dietary Reference Values: A Guide*, Department of Health, 1991

Photographs courtesy of:

Martin Sookias pp 12, 13, 14, 15, 16, 21, 23, 29, 32, 39, 40, 41, 44, 47, 49, 57, 64, 70, 73, 82, 84, 87, 89 (top, middle); **Alamy** pp 61, 63; **Malou Burger** / **FoodDrink** www.foodanddrinkphotos.com p 93; **Food Standards Agency** pp 9, 99; **Fotolia** pp 10 (top), 27, 36, 38, 46, 50, 60, 67, 69 (top, middle, bottom); Bernard BAILLY/Fotolia p 60 (banner); Spurious/Fotolia p 32 (banner); **iStock** pp 8 (banner), 10 (bottom), 11, 43, 59, 62, 86, 92 (banner), 98; eva serrabassa/Istock p 78 (banner); **Science Photo Library**: Oscar Burriel / Science Photo Library p 7; David Mack / Science Photo Library p 77; Philippe Psaila / Science Photo Library p 72; Victor de Schwanberg / Science Photo Library p 31; Petr Jilek/Shutterstock p 44 (banner); **The Advertising Archives** p 75; **The Vegetarian Society** www.vegsoc.org p 89 (bottom)

Front cover photograph courtesy of Jim Wileman

Every effort has been made to trace the copyright holders, but if any have been inadvertently overlooked the publishers will be pleased to make the necessary arrangements at the first opportunity.

Contents

Introduction 4

UNIT ONE

1 Nutrition, diet and health 7

1.1 Introduction to nutrition 1 8
1.2 Introduction to nutrition 2 10
1.3 Introduction to nutrition 3 12
1.4 Macronutrients 1 14
1.5 Macronutrients 2 16
1.6 Macronutrients 3 18
1.7 Micronutrients 1 20
1.8 Micronutrients 2 22
1.9 Diet and health 24
1.10 Energy from foods 26
1.11 Digestion and absorption of nutrients 28

2 Nutritional, physical, chemical and sensory properties of food 31

2.1 Introduction to the effect of storage on nutrients 32
2.2 Food preparation and cooking 1 34
2.3 Food preparation and cooking 2 36
2.4 Food additives 1 38
2.5 Food additives 2 40

3 Techniques and skills in food storage, preparation and cooking 43

3.1 Food storage 44
3.2 Food preparation and cooking 1 46
3.3 Food preparation and cooking 2 48
3.4 Cooking methods 1 50
3.5 Cooking methods 2 52
3.6 Recipe balance and modification 54
3.7 Convenience foods 56

4 Factors affecting consumer choice 59

4.1 Social factors affecting food choice 60
4.2 Economic factors affecting food choice 62
4.3 Factors affecting meal planning 1 64
4.4 Factors affecting meal planning 2 66
4.5 Purchase of food 68
4.6 Choosing large kitchen equipment 70
4.7 Consumer issues and advertising 1 72
4.8 Consumer issues and advertising 2 74

5 Food hygiene and safety 77

5.1 Food spoilage organisms 78
5.2 Food poisoning organisms 80
5.3 Safer food procedures 1 82
5.4 Safer food procedures 2 84
5.5 Food packaging 86
5.6 Food labelling 88

UNIT TWO

6 Controlled Assessment 91

6.1 How Controlled Assessment works 91
6.2 Individual Investigation 92
6.3 Research Task 94
6.4 Primary research methods 96
6.5 Secondary research methods 99

Examination-style questions 101
Glossary 106
Index 110
Acknowledgements 112

Nelson Thornes and AQA

Nelson Thornes has worked in partnership with AQA to make sure that this book offers you the best possible support for your GCSE course. All the content has been approved by the senior examining team at AQA, so you can be sure that it gives you just what you need when you are preparing for your exams.

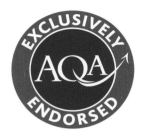

■ How to use this book

This book covers everything you need for your course.

Learning Objectives

At the beginning of each section or topic you'll find a list of Learning Objectives based on the requirements of the specification, so you can make sure you are covering everything you need to know for the exam.

> **Objectives**
> **Objectives**
> **Objectives**
> **Objectives**
> First objective.
> Second objective.

AQA Examiner's Tips

Don't forget to look at the AQA Examiner's Tips throughout the book to help you with your study and prepare for your exam.

> **AQA Examiner's tip**
> Don't forget to look at the AQA Examiner's Tips throughout the book to help you with your study and prepare for your exam.

AQA Examination-style Questions

These offer opportunities to practise doing questions in the style that you can expect in your exam so that you can be fully prepared on the day.

AQA examination questions are reproduced by permission of the Assessment and Qualifications Alliance.

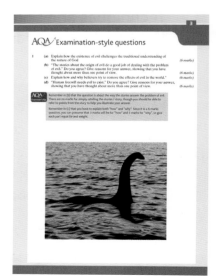

Visit **www.nelsonthornes.com/aqagcse** for more information.

What is Food and Nutrition?

Home Economics: Food and Nutrition is an interesting and stimulating programme of study for students of all ability ranges. The course aims to develop practical food preparation skills and to foster an understanding of the importance of good nutrition and a healthy diet. You will study the scientific processes involved when food is cooked, and how storage and food preparation methods can affect the finished results. The practical cookery skills and theoretical knowledge acquired from this course will equip young people with the ability to make discriminating consumer choices about food and health.

Food and Nutrition involves a study of:

- nutrition, diet and health throughout life.
- nutritional, physical, chemical and sensory properties of food in storage, preparation and cooking.
- techniques and skills in food storage, preparation and cooking.
- factors affecting consumer choice.
- food hygiene and safety.

GCSE Home Economics: Food and Nutrition focuses on practical cookery and all the different ways in which raw ingredients can be made into interesting, healthy and creative dishes which are suitable for a wide variety of situations. This can range from planning and making a simple packed lunch to designing a day's menus for someone with a special dietary need. Alongside the development of practical skills you will study the most recent recommendations for a healthy diet and apply these guidelines when planning practical work and managing resources. Food hygiene and consumer choice are also included as important aspects of this course.

GCSE Home Economics: Food and Nutrition is made up of two units of work:

Unit 1

Written external examination paper, which comprises 40% of the total mark. This is a 1 hour 30 minutes examination paper, which is marked out of 100.

Unit 2

Controlled Assessment (used to be called Coursework) which comprises 60% of the total mark, and is marked out of 160. There are two parts to the Controlled Assessment: an Individual Investigation of 18 hours duration, and a Research Task of 6-8 hours duration. There is more information on the Controlled Assessment in Chapter 6 of this book.

The Controlled Assessment tasks in this book are designed to help you prepare for the tasks your teacher will give to you. The tasks in this book are not designed to test you formally and you cannot use them as your own Controlled Assessment tasks for AQA. Your teacher will not be able to give you as much help with your tasks for AQA as we have given with the tasks in this book.

Home Economics: Food and Nutrition will enable you to develop a wide range of skills. You will:

- actively engage in the subject to develop as effective and independent learners
- develop communication and organisational skills
- develop knowledge and understanding of relevant technological and scientific developments
- develop knowledge and understanding of human needs within a diverse society
- evaluate choices and decisions to develop as informed and discerning consumers.

What is this book about?

This book has been written to support your studies for *GCSE Home Economics: Food and Nutrition* and to enable you to achieve your potential in both the theory examination and the Controlled Assessment.

It is written in student-friendly language and closely follows the five sections of the AQA specification. Each chapter aims to give relevant information on specific topics with activities and questions designed to reinforce the theoretical information provided. Most topics have useful weblinks and Examiner's tips. There are examples of examination-style questions at the end of Chapter 6 which can be used for revision or homework questions. Chapter 6 gives detailed information and advice on methods of research and presentation for the Individual Investigation and the Research task with examples of students' work.

Hopefully this book will provide you with the knowledge and skills needed for a successful outcome in your GCSE examination, but will also develop a lifelong interest in the relationship between food choices and health.

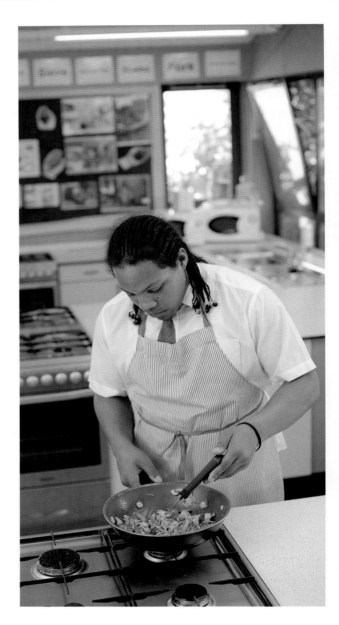

1 Nutrition, diet and health

In this chapter:

1.1–1.3 Introduction to nutrition

1.4–1.6 Macronutrients

1.7–1.8 Micronutrients

1.9 Diet and health

1.10 Energy from foods

1.11 Digestion and absorption of nutrients

To keep fit and healthy we need to understand the importance of the food we eat and how that food is used for growth and maintenance of body cells, to provide energy, and to protect us from ill health.

Foods are made up of nutrients, and learning about these is the study of nutrition. The examination course you are following is called 'Food and Nutrition', so the study of the functions and sources of nutrients is a very important part of the course.

In this chapter you will learn about:

- the study of nutrients and their functions, sources and effects on the body
- the application of nutritional knowledge to the special dietary needs of different population groups
- dietary analysis
- functions of macronutrients in the growth and repair of body cells, and in providing energy and fat-soluble vitamins
- the main food sources for proteins, fats and carbohydrates
- functions of micronutrients in regulating body processes and protecting against infection
- the main food sources for vitamins and minerals
- current nutritional advice and its role in the formation of good eating habits in a multicultural society
- the dietary reference values (DRV) for different population groups
- energy balance and ideal weight
- recommended energy intake from proteins, fats and carbohydrates
- the glycemic index of foods
- the digestion and absorption of nutrients.

What you should already know:

✔ You may have covered healthy eating in Year 9, so you will know that we should eat a balanced diet made up of lots of different foods, and not too many sugary, fatty or salty foods.

✔ You may have heard about the 'Five a Day' fruit and vegetable campaign, from the National Health Service, which aims to get us to eat more fruit and vegetables to improve our health.

✔ You may have seen TV programmes about healthy school meals which tried to get schoolchildren to eat healthier meals at lunchtime.

Introduction to nutrition 1

■ What is nutrition?

Nutrition is the study of the **nutrients** found in food and their functions in the body. The food we eat affects our bodies in many ways, so to stay healthy we need to understand the importance of good nutrition.

What are nutrients?

- Nutrients are chemical compounds which form molecules in food.
- Most foods are made up of more than one nutrient, but no individual food provides all the nutrients that are needed by the body.
- For example, some nutrients help us grow and repair our body tissues: these are called proteins. Others give us energy for our normal daily activities: these are called carbohydrates and fats.
- Lastly, we need small amounts of nutrients called vitamins and minerals. These help to protect the body from infection and regulate body processes such as clotting of the blood and release of energy from food.

Why do we need a balanced diet?

- A **balanced diet** is a diet which contains all the nutrients needed for good health in the correct amounts to meet individual needs.
- For example, an active teenager will need more energy foods than a less active elderly person.
- A good way of making sure we eat a balanced diet is to eat a wide variety of foods, including at least five portions of fruit and vegetables a day and not too many sugary, or fatty foods and drinks.

Malnutrition

Malnutrition can occur when not enough food is eaten to meet dietary needs or when too much is eaten, causing obesity.

Diets can become unbalanced for a variety of reasons:

- Eating too much of one type of food and too little of others. For example, too much carbohydrate and fat and not enough protein, vitamins and minerals. If we eat more energy rich foods than we use up in activity the extra energy will be stored as body fat and we may become obese. Whilst a lack of vitamins and minerals in our diets can result in poor resistance to infections.
- In some countries not enough food is available, so the diet is often deficient in certain nutrients. This can cause poor growth in children and deficiency diseases such as beri-beri and pellagra.
- Some people may not eat enough food to meet their dietary needs. This is called **under-nutrition**. It can be caused by not liking certain foods, such as fruit and vegetables, or by intolerances to foods such as dairy products. Food intake may also be restricted because of a condition called anorexia nervosa which causes severe weight loss and under-nutrition.

Objectives

Understand the relationship between nutrition and good health.

Key terms

Nutrients: chemical compounds found in foods, which include proteins, fats, carbohydrates, vitamins and minerals.

Balanced diet: a diet that contains all the nutrients in the correct amounts to meet individual needs.

Malnutrition: lack of food or particular nutrients in the diet, or too much of the wrong kinds of foods, causing obesity.

AQA **Examiner's tip**

You need to learn the key terms listed as they crop up throughout the examination paper and the Controlled Assessment.

∞ **links**

Find out more at:

www.eatwell.gov.uk/healthydiet/eatwellplate

Remember

To stay healthy we need to eat a wide variety of foods, particularly fresh fruit and vegetables.

The eatwell plate

Use the eatwell plate to help you get the balance right. It shows how much of what you eat should come from each food group.

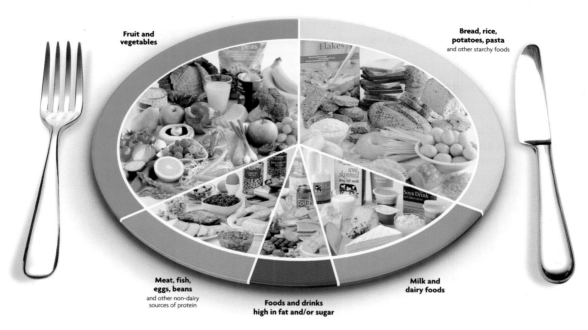

 The eatwell plate

The eatwell plate from the Food Standards Agency (FSA) shows us how much to eat from each food group to stay healthy. You can see that about one third of our food should be from fruits and vegetables; one third from bread, rice, potatoes and pasta; and the rest from milk and dairy foods; and from meat, fish, eggs and beans. Only a very small amount of our intake should be from foods that are high in fat and sugar. Eating a balanced diet that contains a variety of fresh foods helps us stay healthy.

- Elderly people may suffer from under-nutrition if they lose interest in food or are not able to cook for themselves.
- Under-nutrition can cause many health problems such as depression, anaemia, and weak bones and teeth.

Investigation

- Plan a well balanced packed lunch for yourself including foods from each of the five groups shown in the eatwell plate.
- Give reasons why you have chosen each of these items.

Questions

1. What are nutrients?
2. List the **five** main nutrient groups needed for a balanced diet.
3. Why do we need a balanced diet?
4. What is malnutrition?
5. What health problems can be caused by under-nutrition?

Summary

A healthy diet is one that includes the right amounts of proteins, fats, carbohydrates, vitamins and minerals to meet our energy and growth needs.

If we eat more food than we use up in activity we will become overweight.

Introduction to nutrition 2

■ Why do people have different nutritional needs?

Our individual nutritional requirements are determined by our age, gender, activity levels, lifestyle and special needs such as pregnancy or illness.

Factors which affect nutritional requirements

Age

From birth until adulthood the body needs increasing amounts of nutrients for growth and to provide energy for everyday activities. Growth is most rapid from birth to five and during the teenage years. The diet during these growth spurts should provide adequate amounts of: protein for growth; calcium and vitamin D for the formation of healthy bones and teeth; and iron and vitamin C for red blood cells and to prevent anaemia in girls. Teenagers who take part in active sports will also need more energy giving foods.

Once the body is fully grown, metabolism slows down and nutrients are needed to repair and maintain the body and help protect us from infection. As we grow older, and less active, energy requirements decrease, but we still need a good supply of: protein to repair body cells; calcium and vitamin D to prevent brittle bones; and vitamin C to help resist infections.

Gender

Males generally need more energy from foods than females. This is because males have a higher metabolic rate and more muscle tissue.

Physical activity level (PAL)

PAL levels vary depending on work and leisure activities. For example, someone with a sedentary job (mostly sitting down) who does not exercise will have a lower PAL rate than someone with an active job who plays a lot of sport.

Pregnancy and breastfeeding

Pregnant women need to increase their intake of protein, vitamin B (particularly folic acid), vitamins D and C, and calcium, in order to keep themselves and their baby healthy. They do not need to increase their energy intake as they are generally less active and their metabolic rate is slower, particularly during the last few months of pregnancy.

However, breastfeeding mothers do need to increase their energy intake as their food has to supply the energy needs of the baby through breast milk, in addition to their own needs.

Babies

From birth to about six months old, babies should be fed only breast or formula milk as their digestive systems are not able to cope with solid foods. Once they reach six months, solid foods can be introduced gradually along with their milk feeds. This process of introducing solid foods is called weaning.

Key terms

Individual nutritional requirements: the amount of nutrients needed to maintain good health based on age, gender, physical activity and state of health.

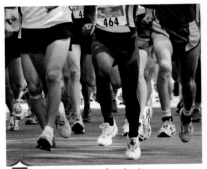

A *Carbohydrate foods give us energy*

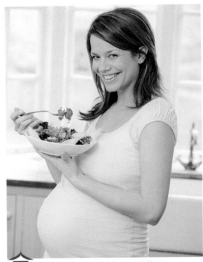

B *Women have slightly different nutritional needs during pregnancy*

AQA *Examiner's tip*

Research different lifestyles so that you can apply the information to different nutritional needs.

From six months old the baby should be eating a variety of solid foods along with most of its milk feeds. Ready prepared weaning foods can be bought in jars or packets, but it is easy to prepare suitable foods by sieving or puréeing foods such as cooked vegetables, fruits and pasta. The texture of weaning foods should be smooth, without lumps, and no salt or sugar should be added. A variety of flavours and textures can gradually be introduced, as long as the foods are salt and sugar free.

By the time babies reach the age of 18 months they should be eating small portions of family meals.

Illness and recovery from operations

The need for different nutrients will vary depending on the type of illness or injury a person has suffered. For example, someone with a bone fracture may need extra calcium and protein; or where blood has been lost, through injury or operation for example, extra iron may be required. A person who is ill may only have a small appetite so the food served should contain protein, and vitamins and minerals with only small amounts of fat and carbohydrate: chicken and vegetable soup, for example.

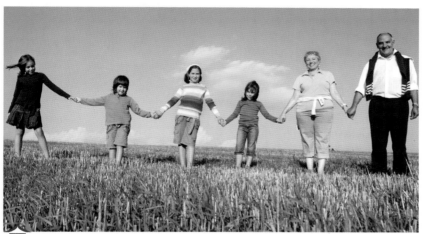

C *Different nutritional needs*

∞links

For more information on weaning please see nhs website:

www.healthystart.nhs.uk

Questions

1. Why do some people require different amounts of nutrients to others?

2. Why do males need more energy foods than females?

3. How does age affect nutritional needs?

4. What is meant by PAL?

5. Which nutrients should be included in the diet of someone recovering from a broken leg?

6. Why do pregnant and breastfeeding women need to increase their intake of certain nutrients?

Summary

People at different life stages need different amounts of nutrients.

Age, gender and physical activity levels (PAL) affect the amounts of nutrients needed by the body.

Pregnant women need to increase their intake of protein, folic acid, vitamins D and C, and calcium.

Dietary analysis

Dietary analysis, using food tables in books or computer programs, is useful as it highlights deficiencies or excesses in a person's nutrient intake. It is a useful tool for carrying out primary research (see 6.4) for investigations into special dietary needs or food related diseases.

Is your diet healthy?

In order to find out if your diet provides adequate amounts of all the nutrients required you should keep a **dietary diary** for at least three days, including one weekend day. This is because we often eat different foods or meals at the weekend.

You should list everything you eat or drink for the three days, including snacks and drinks. You should also record the amount you eat or the size of the portion. For example: a small, medium or large bowl of cereal with semi-skimmed milk; a large jacket potato with two tablespoons of tuna mayonnaise; and a large glass of fresh orange juice. You should also give the number and type: for example, three large slices of granary bread or six roast potatoes.

If you are calculating the nutrient content using a food table book, the weight of different portion sizes can be checked in a book called *Food Portion Sizes* by Helen Crawley (available from H.M.S.O.). Most computer programs used for nutritional analysis will calculate the portion size for you.

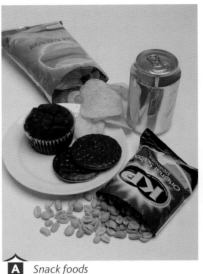

A   *Snack foods*

Key terms

Dietary diary: a record of all the food and drink intake of a person over a given period of days.

AQA **Examiner's tip**

Dietary diaries are only a guide to an individual's food intake as they depend on how accurately they have been recorded. When drawing conclusions on the analysis of dietary diaries remember to make allowances for any inaccuracies in recording.

Remember

When using computer programs to calculate nutritional content, make sure you analyse and interpret the data.

Investigation 1

- Keep a three day dietary record for yourself, using a table like the one below.
- Carry out dietary analysis using a nutritional analysis program or food tables.
- Compare the nutrient intake of your diet with the recommended DRVs for your age group.
- Suggest ways in which your diet might be improved.

B

Day 1	Foods eaten	Amounts
Breakfast	orange juice	large glass / 125 ml
	cornflakes	medium bowl / 30 g
	semi-skimmed milk	1 cup / 100 ml
Lunch		
Evening meal		
Snacks		

Investigation 2 🔍

Using a nutritional analysis program, analyse this sample of a day's food intake of a 15 year old schoolgirl.

Breakfast
- medium glass of fresh orange juice
- 2 Weetabix® with semi-skimmed milk
- 1 large banana

Mid morning
- medium chocolate muffin
- small glass water

Lunch
- 1 large jacket potato with cheddar cheese
- small portion baked beans
- 1 medium sultana flapjack
- small carton of apple juice

Afternoon snack
- bag of salt and vinegar crisps
- small can of diet coke

Evening meal
- medium portion of vegetable curry with rice
- small bowl of vanilla ice cream with 3 tinned peach slices

Snacks
- 2 chocolate digestive biscuits
- small bag of roasted salted peanuts

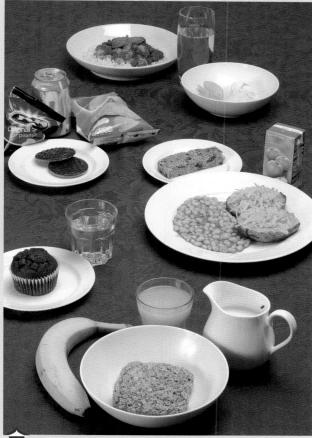

C   *A day's food intake for a 15 year old girl*

Questions

1   Why is dietary analysis useful?

2   List the rules to follow when completing dietary diaries.

3   Why is it useful to include a weekend day in a dietary diary?

Summary

Dietary analysis is a method of assessing the nutritional value of meals.

You can check to see if your diet is lacking in any nutrients by keeping a dietary diary and analysing it using a nutritional analysis program.

1.4 Macronutrients 1

What are macronutrients?

These are nutrients needed by the body in fairly large amounts.

They include **proteins**, fats and carbohydrates.

Why do we need protein foods?

Protein foods are needed for growth, maintenance and repair of all body cells.

Excess protein is converted into glucose and stored in the liver as glycogen which can be used as a secondary source of energy.

Protein molecules are made up of long chains of **amino acids**. There are approximately **22** known amino acids of which **10** are essential for growth and repair in children and **8** are essential for adults. These essential amino acids are sometimes called **indispensable amino acids** because we cannot live without them.

Different proteins are made up of different combinations of amino acids. To stay healthy our bodies need a diet containing a wide variety of protein foods.

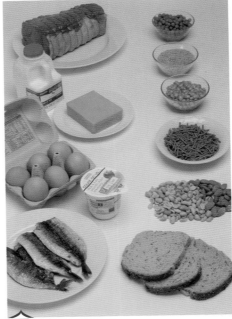

A Protein foods

B Protein values of different foods

Animal proteins	Protein per 100 g	Vegetable proteins	Protein per 100 g
Red meat	25 g	Cereals such as wheat, rice, oats	12 g
Chicken	23 g	Pulses (peas, beans, lentils)	7 g
Fish	20 g	Nuts	11 g
Eggs	12 g	Tofu	8 g
Cheese	26 g	Soya protein (TVP)	16 g
Milk	3.5 g	Quorn™	12 g

Source: adapted from Food Tables, *by A E Bender & D A Bender*

Is there a difference between animal and vegetable sources of protein?

- Animal proteins contain all of the indispensable amino acids. These are sometimes called high biological value (HBV) proteins.
- Vegetable proteins lack one or more of the indispensable amino acids. These are sometimes called low biological value (LBV) proteins.

Does it matter which type of proteins we eat?

Not if we mix and match the protein foods we eat together. For example, a peanut butter sandwich will give us different amino acids in the bread to those in the peanut butter. This is known as complementation of protein and can be used in many different ways: for example, cheese on toast, or hummus and pitta bread. Vegetarians can make sure that they get all the essential amino acids by eating different vegetable protein foods together.

Novel proteins

Novel proteins are grown from micro-organisms which produce mycoprotein, known as Quorn™. It is manufactured into chunks and mince and can be used in pies, sausages, burgers and ready meals. Quorn™ is low in fat, has no cholesterol and is a good source of protein for vegetarians.

How much protein do we need to eat each day?

- Adult females need approximately 45 g per day.
- Adult males need approximately 55 g per day.
- Pregnant women need approximately 51 g per day.
- Breastfeeding women need approximately 56 g per day.

Deficiency

Deficiency is very rare in the UK. In countries that suffer from famine, protein deficiency results in retarded growth in children and wasting of muscles and internal organs.

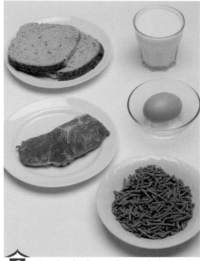

C   *Foods which supply our daily intake of protein*

Questions

1. What are macronutrients?

2. Why is protein needed by the body?

3. What is protein made up of?

4. What is the nutritional difference between animal and vegetable proteins?

5. Why do some people need more proteins than others?

6. Give examples of how protein foods can be combined to complement each other.

7. What are novel proteins?

Summary

Macronutrients are needed by the body in relatively large amounts.

Proteins, fats and carbohydrates are macronutrients.

Animal proteins contain all the essential amino acids (HBV).

Vegetable proteins lack one or more essential amino acids (LBV).

Fats

Why do we need fats?

Fats provide the body with the most concentrated source of energy and supply the fat-soluble vitamins A, D, E and K. Fats also provide a protective layer around delicate internal organs such as the kidneys.

Composition of fats

- Fats are composed of the elements carbon, oxygen and hydrogen.
- They are made up of one molecule of glycerol and three fatty acids.
- The chemical composition of fats varies according to the number of double bonds in their structure.
- **Saturated fatty acids** have no double bonds, as all the carbon atoms are saturated with hydrogen.
- **Unsaturated fatty acids** have two or more double bonds.
- Monounsaturated fatty acids have one double bond.
- Polyunsaturated fatty acids contain many double bonds.
- Fats containing double bonds are healthier than fats that do not contain double bonds.

Animal fats

These are mostly made up of saturated fatty acids which are converted to cholesterol in the liver. We need some cholesterol for healthy body cells and hormones, but if we eat too much saturated fat the resulting cholesterol can block our arteries and cause heart disease.

Examples of foods containing animal fats are: all meats, including bacon and sausage; pate; suet; eggs; milk, cream and butter. Animal fats are usually solid at room temperature.

Vegetable fats

These are mostly made up of unsaturated fatty acids which are not converted into cholesterol and are thought to be healthier than animal fats. People who live in Mediterranean countries, and eat olive oil and fish and very little animal fat, tend to have lower rates of heart disease than people who eat large amounts of animal fat.

Examples of foods containing vegetable fats are: corn, olive and sunflower oils; margarine; nuts and seeds; wholegrain cereals; and avocado pears. Oils are usually liquid at room temperature.

Remember

Fat should provide no more than 35% of total energy and saturated fat no more than 11% of total energy.

Key terms

Saturated fatty acids: from animal food sources – have no double bonds, as all the carbon atoms are saturated with hydrogen.

Unsaturated fatty acids: from vegetable sources – have two or more double bonds.

AQA Examiner's tip

Look at food labels to find out which foods are high in fat. Learn the difference between saturated and unsaturated fats.

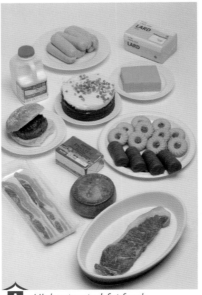
A High saturated fat foods

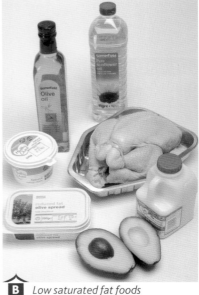
B Low saturated fat foods

Ways of cutting down on saturated fat

- Reduce the amount of fried foods eaten, including chips.
- Cut all visible fat off meat and bacon.
- Eat more chicken and fish and less red meat.
- Eat low fat spreads, cheese and yoghurts.
- Use an oil spray or a nonstick frying pan to reduce the amount of fat used in cooking.
- Buy lean mince and low fat sausages.
- Cut down on cakes, biscuits and pastries.
- Reduce the fat content in recipes when baking.

Practical activity

- Plan and make a selection of dishes to show how recipes can be adapted to either reduce the fat content, or to swap saturated fats for unsaturated fats.
- Photograph your results and make a chart for a class display.

C *Uses of fats in cooking*

Type of fat	Production method	Uses in cooking
Hard or block margarine	• Made from different animal and vegetable fats which are hardened by a process called hydrogenation.	• Adds colour to pastry, scones and biscuits. • Useful for rubbed-in mixture, as it does not go oily when handled.
Soft margarine	• Made from vegetable oils which have been hydrogenated and emulsified. • It is not hydrogenated as much as hard margarine and is softer in texture.	• Used for spreading on bread etc. • Suitable for creaming methods.
Low fat spread	• This is made in the same way as soft margarine but contains added water which reduces the fat content.	• Used mainly for spreading. • Some claim that they can be used for baking and frying.
Butter	• Made by churning cream from milk. • Butter must be at least 82 % fat and is high in saturates.	• Used in cooking to give extra flavour to pastry and biscuits. • Can be used for sauces. • Used for spreading on bread etc.
Ghee	• Clarified unsalted butter.	• Used in curries and sauces.
Lard	• Made from rendered pig fat. • It is a solid saturated fat.	• Used to give a crumbly texture to shortcrust pastry. • Can be used for frying. • Vegetarians and some religious groups will not use lard.
Suet	• Made from the shredded fatty tissues found round the internal organs of animals.	• Used in suet pastry, dumplings and some Christmas puddings. • Vegetarians will not eat suet.
Oils	• Vegetable and fish oils are liquid at room temperature. • They are refined and bottled, ready for use.	• Used in salad dressings. • Can be used for frying and roasting. • Can be used in some baked recipes such as bread.
White vegetable fat	• Made from emulsified vegetable oils such as sunflower oil. • Low in saturated fat and a healthier alternative to lard.	• Can be used for making pastry. • Can be used for frying and roasting. • Suitable for vegetarians.

Questions

1. Why are fats needed by the body?
2. What is the difference between animal and vegetable fats?
3. Why are saturated fats less healthy than unsaturated fats?

Summary

Fats are the most concentrated source of energy and provide fat-soluble vitamins.

Saturated fats are from animal sources such as meat and dairy products.

Unsaturated fats are from vegetable sources such as sunflower oil, nuts and seeds.

Carbohydrates

Why do we need carbohydrates?

Carbohydrate foods are needed to provide energy. Carbohydrates, in particular starchy foods, are the cheapest source of energy and are easily digested. When carbohydrate foods such as bread, pasta and potatoes are eaten they are broken down into glucose during digestion and absorbed into the bloodstream to be used for energy. Excess glucose is stored in the liver as glycogen and can be used when extra energy is needed.

Carbohydrates eaten with proteins allow the proteins to be used for growth and repair rather than for energy. As protein foods are usually more expensive than carbohydrates this is sometimes called **protein sparing**.

Carbohydrates should provide 50 per cent of the total energy intake, with no more than 11 per cent from sugars.

If too much carbohydrate is eaten, and it is not needed for energy or glycogen stores, it is stored as body fat.

Main food sources

Carbohydrates can be divided into three main groups: sugars, starches and **dietary fibre** or **non-starch polysaccharide (NSP)**.

Objectives

Understand the function of carbohydrates in the provision of energy.

Key terms

Non-starch polysaccharide (NSP), also known as dietary fibre: the indigestible fibrous structure of plants. It is not a nutrient, but is essential for the elimination of waste products from the large intestine.

AQA Examiner's tip

Make sure you are familiar with high fibre foods and ways in which sugar can be reduced in recipes.

A Food sources of sugars, starches and NSP

Intrinsic sugars (sometimes called natural sugars)	Extrinsic sugars (added sugars)	Starches	Non-starch polysaccharide (NSP) (dietary fibre)
• Form part of the cell structure of plants in some fruits and vegetables. • **Fructose**: found in fruit and honey. • **Glucose**: found in ripe fruits and some vegetables such as onions and beetroot. • **Galactose**: found in milk as part of the milk sugar lactose. • **Lactose**: found in milk and milk products.	• Not part of the cell structure of plants, but are added to foods to provide sweetness and a quick source of energy. • **Sucrose**: obtained by refining cane sugar or sugar beet. • This is the sugar that is used in recipes or added to drinks. • No food value other than providing a quick source of energy, so sometimes referred to as 'empty' calories. • **Honey**: obtained from honeycomb produced by bees.	• Formed from long chains of glucose units. • Produced during photosynthesis in plants. • Take longer to digest than sugars so release energy more slowly into the bloodstream and over a longer period of time. • Sometimes referred to as slow releasing carbohydrates.	• Found in the cell structure of plants in the form of cellulose and pectin. • Humans cannot digest dietary fibre, but it is very important in moving waste materials in the large intestine. • Dietary fibre can also help to control blood sugar levels. Foods rich in dietary fibre can help us to feel full for longer, so we are less likely to snack on sugary foods. • Foods containing dietary fibre are also low in fat and contain valuable vitamins and minerals.
Sources Fruit, onions, tomatoes, beetroot, milk	**Sources** Sucrose is refined from sugar cane and sugar beet into granulated, castor, and demerara sugar; and golden syrup. Honey is obtained from honeycomb and undergoes various degrees of refinement.	**Sources** Cereals, bread, root vegetables, pulses (peas, beans and lentils), bananas, rice, pasta	**Sources** Pulses (beans, peas and lentils), wholemeal bread, wholegrain cereals, wholewheat pasta, brown rice, baked potato with skin, dried fruits (including apricots, dates and figs), all vegetables

B *Types of carbohydrate and uses in cooking*

Type of carbohydrate	Production method	Uses in cooking
Wheat	• Flour is produced from cereals by a process called milling, which creates a fine powder. • The flour is sieved to remove the bran and husk. • Wholemeal flour contains the bran, which provides dietary fibre in wholemeal produce.	• Wheat flour can be plain, self-raising or wholemeal. • Used for bread, biscuits, cakes and pastries.
Oats	• Oats are rolled to produce flakes. • Can be sold as oatmeal which is more finely rolled. • Oats are high in dietary fibre and may help to reduce cholesterol in the blood.	• Breakfast cereals such as muesli and porridge. • Flapjacks, cakes and biscuits. • Oatmeal can also be used for coating fish.
Rice	• Rice is a cereal plant and is milled after harvesting to remove the husk. • It can be crushed and made into ground rice.	Two main types of rice are: • long grain (or patna) – usually boiled and served with savoury dishes such as curries. • short grain – used for puddings and rice cakes.
Maize (sweetcorn)	• Grains are crushed and made into a flour or refined to make cornflour.	• Cobs can be boiled and eaten as a vegetable. • Maize flour is used to make tortillas. • Cornflour is pure starch and is used as a thickening agent.
Pasta	• Pasta is produced from durum wheat flour, which is mixed with water, oil and sometimes egg, to produce a dough that can be rolled and cut to various shapes.	• Usually boiled and served with meat, fish or vegetable sauces or made into dishes such as lasagne.
Potatoes and other root vegetables	• Potatoes and root vegetables are a good source of carbohydrate in the diet and can be used fresh or dried.	• Can be boiled, roasted, fried or baked; and used in soups, curries and casseroles.
Sugar (sucrose)	• Refined sugar is made from crushing, milling and sieving sugar cane or sugar beet. • Brown sugar is the least refined. • White sugar has been refined to remove all of the coloured residue.	• Brown sugar is used for coffee; for baking gingerbread and flapjacks; and making toffee and syrups. • White sugar is used in baking cakes, biscuits and pastry.

Investigation

- Look in a recipe book and find one sweet and one savoury recipe that you could alter to increase the dietary fibre content.
- Use a nutritional analysis program to work out the dietary fibre content of the original recipe and your adapted version.
- Comment on your results, making reference to the DRVs for dietary fibre.

Questions

1   Why do we need carbohydrates in our diets?

2   What are the three groups of carbohydrates?

3   What is the difference between intrinsic and extrinsic sugars?

4   What is dietary fibre?

5   Why is it important in our diets?

6   List the foods that are good sources of dietary fibre.

Summary

The three types of carbohydrates are sugars, starches and non-starch polysaccharide (NSP), also known as dietary fibre.

Starchy carbohydrates, such as bread and potatoes, are the healthiest sources of energy in the diet.

Wholegrain carbohydrates, such as cereals, provide the body with dietary fibre.

1.7 Micronutrients 1

What are micronutrients?

Micronutrients are vitamins and minerals. These are nutrients which are needed in smaller quantities than the macronutrients (see 1.4–1.6) and are used by the body for protection from infection, and to regulate body processes such as the absorption of energy from food.

Vitamins

Vitamins can be divided into **water soluble vitamins** (those which dissolve in water) and **fat-soluble vitamins**. Water soluble vitamins cannot be stored in the body and need to be eaten every day. Most fat-soluble vitamins can be stored in the liver so do not have to be eaten every day.

Objectives

Understand the functions and food sources of micronutrients in our diet.

Key terms

Water soluble vitamins: vitamins B and C dissolve in water.

Fat-soluble vitamins: vitamins A, D, E and K are present in the fat content of foods.

A *Functions and sources of water soluble vitamins*

Vitamin	Function	Sources	Deficiency
B_1 (thiamin)	• Releases energy from carbohydrates. • Promotes healthy nervous system.	Fortified flours and breakfast cereals; yeast extract; meat (especially pork); milk, cheese, and eggs; peas and potatoes	• Loss of appetite, fatigue and dizziness. • Slow growth in children. • Severe deficiencies can cause beri-beri.
B_2 (riboflavin)	• Promotes healthy skin and mouth. • Releases energy to body cells.	Liver and kidney; breakfast cereals; yeast extract; cheese, eggs and milk; wholemeal bread; potatoes and cabbage	• Cracks around mouth and lips. • Tongue and eyes may become inflamed. • General tiredness.
B_3 (nicotinic acid)	• Releases energy from carbohydrates, fats and proteins.	A wide range of foods including: all meat; tuna; yeast extract; beef extract; bread; cheese; potatoes	• Skin problems such as dermatitis. • Severe deficiency causes pellagra but this is very rare in the UK.
B_{12} (cyanocobalamin)	• Helps prevent anaemia. • Promotes healthy nervous system.	Liver, meat and fish; cheese, milk and eggs; fortified breakfast cereals	• Anaemia. • Strict vegetarians may suffer from deficiencies, as B_{12} is mostly found in animal products.
Folic acid (folate)	• Helps to prevent premature birth and neural tube defects during pregnancy. • Needed for the formation of red blood cells.	Broccoli, cabbage, spinach, cress and rocket leaves; bread; potatoes; yeast extract; nuts and seeds; breakfast cereals	• Tiredness. • Anaemia. • Pregnant women should take a folic acid supplement during the first half of pregnancy to prevent birth defects.
C (ascorbic acid)	• Needed for formation of connective tissue, bone and tooth enamel. • Helps absorb iron into the blood. • Needed for the healing of wounds and fractures. • An antioxidant vitamin.	Green vegetables and potatoes; citrus fruits and blackcurrants	• Mouth and gum infections. • Slow healing of wounds and fractures. • Extreme deficiency causes scurvy but this is almost unknown in the UK.

Investigation 🔍

■ Plan a day's meals that would provide a good supply of folic acid for a pregnant woman.

■ Analyse your meals using a nutritional analysis program and evaluate your results.

B *Functions and sources of fat-soluble vitamins*

Vitamin	Function	Sources	Deficiency
A (retinol) (animal sources)	• Needed for healthy mucous membranes in nose, throat and digestive system. • Needed for formation of visual purple in the eye which helps us to see in dim light.	Milk and cheese; eggs; oily fish and cod liver oil; liver and kidney	• Poor eyesight or night blindness. • But deficiency is rare in the UK as vitamin A is found in a wide variety of foods. • Excess in pregnancy can cause birth defects. Pregnant women are advised not to eat liver, as it contains large amounts of retinol.
A (beta-carotene) (vegetable sources)	• Beta-carotene is an antioxidant vitamin.	Carrots, spinach, tomatoes and broccoli; apricots; fortified margarines	
D (choleocalciferol)	• Promotes the absorption of calcium to form healthy bones and teeth.	Fish liver oils and oily fish; eggs, cheese and butter; fortified margarines; the action of sunlight on the skin	• Deficiency can cause rickets in children and brittle bones in older people. • Both of these conditions can be prevented by exposure to sunlight.
E (tocopherols)	• Needed for healthy skin and reproductive system. • An antioxidant vitamin.	Most plant foods and vegetable oils; eggs; cereal products	• Deficiency very rare. • No evidence that vitamin E delays ageing.
K	• Needed for normal clotting of the blood.	Green leafy vegetables such as spinach and cabbage; meat and liver	• Deficiency is rare when a varied diet is eaten.

Source: Bender AE & Bender DA, Food Tables, *1986*

Antioxidant vitamins

The antioxidant vitamins protect body cells from damage and help to reduce the risk of cancer and heart disease. They are:

Vitamin A

This is in the form of beta-carotenes which are found in orange and dark coloured vegetables and fruits. These include: sweet potatoes, carrots, tomatoes, apricots, peaches, mango, spinach and broccoli.

Vitamin C

Vitamin C (ascorbic acid) is plentiful in our diets if we eat at least five portions of fruit and vegetables a day. Most people in this country get a large amount of vitamin C from potatoes as we tend to eat them every day. Other good sources of vitamin C include: fresh orange juice, blackcurrant juice, broccoli and tomatoes.

Vitamin E

Foods rich in vitamin E include: vegetable oils, such as sunflower and wheatgerm, nuts, cereal products and eggs.

C *Foods which supply antioxidant vitamins*

> **Remember**
>
> ACE = antioxidant vitamins which may protect the body from heart disease and cancer.

> **AQA** *Examiner's tip*
>
> When answering questions on micronutrients, make sure you name the vitamin to get maximum marks.

> **Summary**
>
> Micronutrients are vitamins and minerals.
>
> They are only needed in very small amounts in our diets, but are vital for good health.

Minerals

Minerals are used by the body for:

- building strong bones and teeth
- forming healthy blood cells and carrying oxygen around the body
- controlling body processes such as nerve impulses
- regulating body fluids.

Some minerals are needed in fairly large amounts and these include **calcium** and **iron**. Others are only needed in very small amounts and are known as **trace elements**, which include fluoride and iodine.

Are you getting enough calcium?

Calcium is a very important mineral for everyone, as it is used to build strong bones and teeth and to protect us from bone diseases in later life. Some research has shown that calcium may also help to reduce high blood pressure and to protect us from some forms of cancer.

To absorb calcium effectively we must also have an adequate supply of vitamin D, which is present in dairy produce and fortified margarine, and is also produced by the action of sunlight on the skin.

Eating a varied diet containing milk, cheese, green vegetables, soya products, nuts and bread should provide you with adequate amounts of calcium.

The recommended amount of calcium for adults is 700 mg per day.

Objectives

Develop knowledge of the function of minerals in the body.

Key terms

Calcium: mineral needed for strong bones and teeth.

Iron: mineral needed for healthy red blood cells and carrying oxygen round the body.

Trace elements: minerals needed in very small amounts in the diet.

AQA Examiner's tip

Look in a book of food tables, for example, *Bender & Bender*, and make a list of the best food sources of calcium and iron.

A *Functions and sources of minerals*

Mineral	Function	Sources	Deficiency
Calcium	• Used to develop strong bones and teeth. • Needed for muscle contraction, blood clotting and a healthy nervous system.	Milk, cheese, butter and yogurt; eggs; sardines; white bread; nuts; cabbage, spinach and oranges	• Weak bones and teeth. • Rickets in children and osteomalacia in adults.
Iron	• Used in formation of haemoglobin in red blood cells which carry oxygen around the body.	Red meat and liver; oily fish; breakfast cereals and wholemeal bread; spinach, cabbage and broccoli; dried fruit; pulses; cocoa powder and plain chocolate	• Can cause tiredness and anaemia. • Menstruating women can be deficient where dietary intakes of iron are low.
Fluoride	• Strengthens teeth by combining with enamel coating, making them more resistant to attack by acids.	Tea; drinking water in areas where fluoride is added; seafood	Deficiency is very rare.
Sodium	• Maintains correct concentration of body fluids.	Table salt; cooked meats; bacon and sausages; canned foods; ready meals; salty snack foods	Deficiency is very rare.
Iodine	• Makes the hormone thyroxine, which is produced by the thyroid gland in the neck. • Used to control the body's metabolism.	Seafood; milk; cod liver oil; green vegetables; tap water; iodised salt	• Slow metabolism. • Enlargement of the thyroid gland causing goitre neck.

Investigation 1

- Make a list of everything you ate and drank yesterday.

- Analyse your list using a nutritional analysis program, or use a book of food tables, to work out the calcium content.

- Compare your totals with the DRVs for calcium for your age group.

- If your diet is low in calcium, make suggestions as to ways in which you could improve it.

Are you getting enough iron?

Iron is essential for making red blood cells which carry oxygen around the body. It is important for everyone to have a varied diet that contains iron rich foods.

There are two main sources of iron: **haem iron**, which is found in meat and is easily absorbed by the body; and **non-haem iron**, which is found in beans, nuts, soya products, wholegrains and fortified breakfast cereals, and is less easily absorbed by the body. Some green vegetables such as watercress, broccoli and curly kale also supply good amounts of non-haem iron.

However, spinach, made popular by 'Popeye the sailor man', is not a good source of iron. This is because, although it contains iron, it also contains phytic acid which makes it harder for the body to absorb the iron. Tea and coffee contain polyphenols, which also reduce the amount of iron absorbed from food, so it is better not to drink tea and coffee with meals.

Vitamin C helps to increase absorption of iron from food so drinking orange juice, or eating fruit and vegetables rich in vitamin C, as part of a meal helps to increase the amount of iron absorbed.

The recommended intake of iron per day is: 8.7 mg for a man, and 14.8 mg for a woman.

Practical activity 1

- Plan and make a main meal for a teenager that would give adequate amounts of calcium and iron.

Practical activity 2

Toddlers and young children need good supplies of calcium for the formation of healthy bones and teeth.

- Plan and cook a selection of items rich in calcium that would be suitable to serve at a three year old's birthday party.

- Analyse the items made, using 'Food for a PC' or a similar nutritional analysis program.

Questions

1   Why is calcium needed by the body?

2   Which group of foods is particularly rich in calcium?

3   Why do we need iron in the diet?

4   Why do teenage girls need good supplies of iron rich foods?

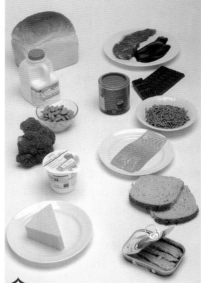

B   *Foods rich in calcium and iron*

Investigation 2

- Follow the link below for information on iron rich meals and snacks.

- Print off the information.

- Analyse the menus using a nutritional analysis program and work out the total iron content of the day's meals.

- Compare the totals with the DRVs for iron for a teenage girl.

- Examine your own diet to find out if you are deficient in iron.

∞ links

Find more information on iron rich meals and snacks at:

www.eatwell.gov.uk/healthissues/irondeficiency

Summary

Adequate amounts of iron and calcium in our diet are vital for good health.

Some minerals, such as iodine and fluoride, are known as trace elements because they are only needed in minute amounts.

1.9 Diet and health

Where do we get current nutritional advice from?

There are different sources of information and advice about nutrition, some are official and others are voluntary.

Official sources of information

- Government reports – for example, COMA report 1991
- Government departments – for example, MAFF Balance of Good Health
- Food Standards Agency – for example, Eatwell Plate and Traffic Light System
- National Health Service – for example, Five a Day campaign
- British Nutrition Foundation – nutrition information
- Schools Food Trust – new standards for school meals

Voluntary sources of information

- Food labels
- Free leaflets
- Media – including TV programmes, magazines, newspapers and books

Healthy eating guidelines advise us to:

- eat less fat, sugar and salt.
- eat more **dietary fibre** and starchy foods.
- eat at least five portions of fruit and vegetables every day.

The Government published these eight tips for eating well in October 2005.

- Base your meals on **starchy foods.**
- Eat lots of fruit and vegetables.
- Eat more fish.
- Cut down on **saturated fats** and sugar.
- Try to eat less salt – no more than 6 g a day.
- Get active and try to be a healthy weight.
- Drink plenty of water.
- Don't skip breakfast.

Why do we need to follow dietary guidelines?

To keep us healthy and prevent dietary related diseases. For example:

- too much fat can lead to obesity and coronary heart disease.
- too much sugar can lead to obesity, diabetes and tooth decay.
- too much salt can lead to hypertension (high blood pressure) and strokes.
- too little dietary fibre can lead to constipation and diverticulitis.

Key terms

Dietary fibre: refers to non-starch polysaccharides which are found in fruit and vegetables.

Starchy foods: cereals, vegetables, fruit, pasta, rice, potatoes and bread.

Saturated fats: fats from animal sources such as meat, eggs, milk, butter and cheese.

Investigation

- Carry out an investigation of a person with a special dietary need, such as someone suffering from diabetes or heart disease.

- Plan a range of healthy dishes that would be suitable for a person suffering from the chosen condition.

- Make up some of the dishes in your practical lessons.

- Carry out a sensory and nutritional analysis of your practical work.

- Evaluate the results of your case study.

How do we know how much of each nutrient we should be eating each day?

Government guidelines for nutrient intakes try to cover a wide range of individual needs but these are only general guidelines for average nutrient requirements.

DRV – Dietary reference value. This is an overall term used to cover EAR, LRNI and RNI.

EAR – Estimated average requirement for any group of people but, like any average, some will need more and some will need less.

RNI – Reference nutrient intake. An amount of a nutrient that is enough, or more than enough, for approximately 97 per cent of a population group.

LRNI – Lower reference nutrient intake is the amount of nutrient that is enough for a few people in a population group who have low needs.

Safe intake – This term is used where there is lack of evidence regarding how much of a nutrient is needed by the body. Safe intake, as its name suggests, is the amount that is thought to satisfy most people's needs without any harmful effects.

GDA – Guideline daily amounts were developed by food manufacturers and retailers. Based on DRVs they are intended to simplify nutritional information on food labels.

AQA Examiner's tip

Learn the DRVs for the main nutrients in your age group.

Questions

1. What are the current dietary guidelines for healthy eating?
2. Where can we get information on healthy eating?

Summary

Government guidelines for nutrient intakes are designed to cover a wide range of individual needs.

DRVs for different nutrients give us a guide to how much of a particular nutrient we should be eating each day.

A *DRVs for 11–18 year olds*

	Males (per day)	Females (per day)
Protein	55.5 g	45 g
Fat	No more than 35 % of total food energy, of which no more than 11 % should be from saturated fat	No more than 35 % of total food energy, of which no more than 11 % should be from saturated fat
Total energy	11–14 years 2220 kcals 15–18 years 2755 kcals	11–14 years 1845 kcals 15–18 years 2110 kcals
Vitamin A	700 µg	600 µg
Vitamin B$_1$ (thiamin)	1 mg	0.9 mg
Vitamin B$_2$ (riboflavin)	1.3 mg	1.1 mg
Vitamin B$_3$ (nicotinic acid)	17 mg	13 mg
Folate	200 µg	200 µg
Vitamin C	35–40 mg	35–40 mg
Vitamin D	No recommendation for school age children	No recommendation for school age children
Vitamin E	Safe intake not more than 4 mg	Safe intake not more than 3 mg
Vitamin K	No DRVs	No DRVs
Minerals Iron	8.7 mg	14.8 mg
Calcium	1000 mg	800 mg
Sodium	1600 mg	1600 mg

Source: For further information on DRVs for other groups, see Dietary Reference Values: A Guide, *Department of Health, 1991*

Energy from foods

Why do we need energy?

We need energy for every bodily process from breathing, blood circulation and brain function, to playing football and dancing. We even need energy when we are sleeping. Different activities require different amounts of energy, and the more active we are the more energy we use up.

Basal metabolic rate (BMR) is the rate at which the body uses energy when it is warm and resting. Energy requirements depend on age, gender and activity levels. More energy is needed during periods of rapid growth such as infancy and teenage years. Less energy is needed once our bodies are fully grown, and even less during middle and old age when we are less active.

Energy giving foods

Energy is provided by the food we eat after it has been digested. The three main nutrients that provide energy are:

- carbohydrates (sugars and starches)
- fats
- proteins.

Carbohydrates, such as bread, pasta, rice and potatoes, are the cheapest sources of energy. They also tend to be low in fat so are healthy options for providing energy.

Fats are said to be **energy dense** as they provide more than twice the amount of kilocalories per gram than carbohydrates or proteins. Fats, in particular saturated fats, are not such a healthy source of energy and fat should not exceed 35 per cent of total energy food intake.

Proteins can provide energy in a diet which is low in carbohydrate, but it is an expensive way of providing energy.

The glycemic index (GI) of foods

This is the rate at which carbohydrates are converted into glucose during digestion.

Foods with a high glycemic index are converted rapidly and give an immediate burst of energy. These foods are usually made from refined sugar or white flour and include most sweets, cakes, biscuits and fizzy drinks.

Low GI foods are converted to glucose more slowly and are sometimes referred to as slow releasing carbohydrates as they provide energy over a longer period of time. These foods include wholegrain products, nuts, seeds, and fruits such as apples and bananas.

Low GI foods are healthier as they help you to feel fuller for longer and control the release of the hormone insulin into the body. They also contain more dietary fibre than high GI foods.

Objectives

Understand energy needs throughout life.

Understand the importance of energy balance in maintaining healthy body weight.

Key terms

Basal metabolic rate (BMR): the rate at which the body uses energy when it is warm and resting.

Energy dense: containing high amounts of fat and sugar.

A DRVs for energy requirements of different age groups

Age	Males (kcals per day)	Females (kcals per day)
0–6 months	690	645
7–12 months	920	865
1–3 years	1230	1165
4–6 years	1715	1545
11–14 years	2220	1845
15–18 years	2755	2110
19–49 years	2550	1940
50–59 years	2550	1900
60–74 years	2330	1900
75 +	2100	1810

Source: Adapted from Dietary Reference Values, Department of Health, 1991

B *Recommended sources of food energy in the UK*

Protein	No more than 15 % of total food energy from protein.	
Carbohydrate	Bulk of food energy (50 %) from carbohydrates.	Most of carbohydrate food energy (39 %) from starch.
		No more than 11 % from non-milk extrinsic sugars.
Fat	No more than 35 % of total food energy from fats.	No more than 11 % of food energy from saturated fats.
		Other sources of energy from fats: 12.1 % monounsaturated fats; 6.5 % polyunsaturated fats and 1.2 % trans fats.

Source: Department of Health, 1991

AQA **Examiner's tip**

Be familiar with the DRVs for energy for your age range. Remember males need more energy than females as they have a higher metabolic rate and burn energy faster than females.

Energy balance

To remain healthy and prevent obesity we must balance the amount of food we eat with the amount of energy we use up in activity. If more food is eaten than is used up as energy it is stored as body fat. To lose weight we need to eat fewer energy dense foods, in particular those high in fat and sugar, and increase our physical activity.

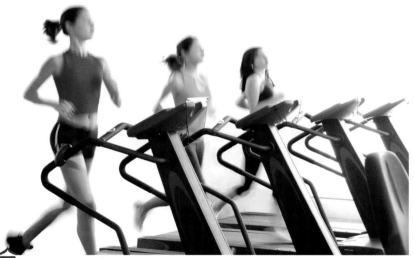

C *Increase physical activity*

Practical activity

- Plan and make a low fat, high energy meal that would be suitable for a teenager to eat before playing football later in the day.
- Calculate the kilocalories per portion from the fat, protein and carbohydrate content of the meal.
- Evaluate your results.

Questions

1. Why do we need energy?

2. What are the energy giving nutrient groups?

3. What is BMR?

4. Look at Table **A** and explain the different energy requirements for different individuals.

5. Why are low GI foods healthier sources of energy than high GI foods?

6. Give **six** examples of low GI foods.

Summary

Energy is needed by the body for every process and activity.

Carbohydrates, fats and proteins provide the body with energy.

Energy balance is when the energy intake of food equals that used up in energy expenditure.

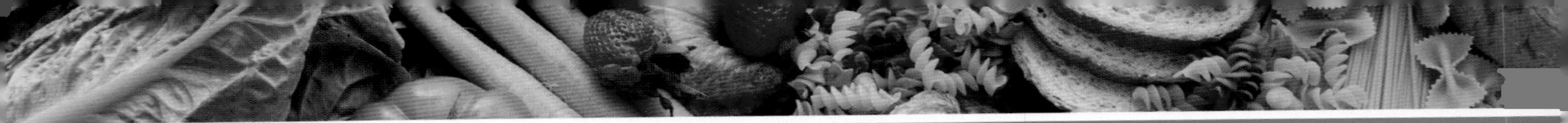

1.11 Digestion and absorption of nutrients

What happens to food once we have eaten it?

To allow the body to use the nutrients in food for energy, growth, repair and protection, the food must be broken down or **digested**.

Digestive process

- Food enters the mouth where it is broken down into smaller pieces by the action of chewing.
- Saliva in the mouth contains a **digestive enzyme** (salivary amylase) which starts to break down cooked starch into sugars.
- When food is swallowed it passes down the oesophagus into the stomach.
- The enzyme pepsin, in the gastric juice of the stomach, starts the digestion of proteins into amino acids.
- The liver produces bile which emulsifies fats.
- Food stays in the stomach for four to five hours where it is moved around by muscular action and mixed with gastric juices.
- Food then passes through the first part of the small intestine (duodenum) where enzymes (proteinase) continue to break down proteins; fat is broken down into fatty acids and glycerol by the enzyme lipase; and carbohydrates are broken down into glucose by the enzyme amylase.
- It then passes into the second part of the small intestine (ileum) where most of the nutrients are absorbed into the bloodstream and carried around the body.
- Finally, the undigested food (including fibre) passes to the large intestine (colon) and is excreted through the anus.

Objectives

Develop outline knowledge of digestion and absorption of nutrients.

Understand the functions of water in the diet.

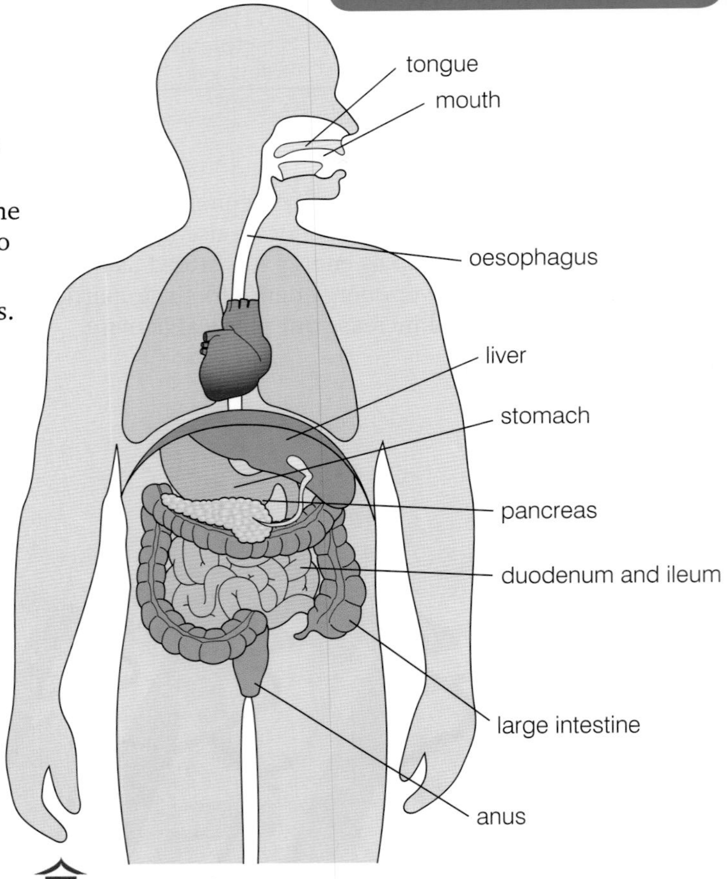

A *The human digestive system*

Water

Almost 70 per cent of the human body is made up of water. Water is needed for:

- body fluids, such as blood, sweat and urine
- regulation of body temperature
- body processes, such as digestion
- preventing dehydration.

Water is lost from the body in urine, faeces and sweat, and through **respiration**. So we need to replace it every day to prevent dehydration.

Key terms

Digestive enzymes: chemicals in the digestive juices which speed up the breakdown of food and the release of nutrients.

Respiration: process in which air passes into and out of the lungs so that the blood can absorb oxygen and give off carbon dioxide and water.

Water in the diet

Many foods such as vegetables and fruit provide water, but we mainly get water from drinks, including fizzy drinks, fruit juices, tea and coffee. Altogether we need about two to three litres a day (the equivalent of six to eight glasses) to stay healthy. Drinking tap water is the best way of making sure we get enough fluids, especially in hot weather when the body loses fluids through sweating. Extra water is also needed during illness where the patient has a high temperature and after strenuous exercise to prevent dehydration.

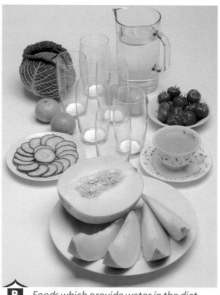

B   *Foods which provide water in the diet*

How does water aid digestion?

Water is needed: to eliminate waste products from the large intestine; to prevent constipation; and to filter impurities from the kidneys, by the production of urine.

Investigation

- Keep a dietary diary of everything you eat and drink in one day.
- Analyse your food intake for the water content, and calculate whether you meet your daily requirement of two to three litres of water a day.

Questions

1. What is the function of saliva in the digestive process?

2. Name the enzyme in the gastric juice that starts the digestion of proteins.

3. Where are most of the nutrients in food absorbed into the bloodstream?

4. Why is water important in the digestive process?

5. Copy Diagram **A** and discuss the digestive process that would be involved after eating a meal of poached egg and wholemeal toast.

Summary

Digestion starts in the mouth where food is broken down by the action of chewing.

Different digestive enzymes work on different nutrients.

Nutrients are absorbed into the bloodstream in the small intestine.

Water is needed to eliminate waste products.

C   *Water content of foods*

Food	Water content (%)
Cucumber	96
Onions	93
Melon	93
Cabbage	90
Strawberries	88
Milk	87.6
Yogurt	79
Bananas	70
Apples	65
Chicken	63
Minced beef	59
Sausages	48
Bread	39
Cheddar cheese	37
Crisps	3

Source: Bender AE & Bender DA, Food Tables, 1986

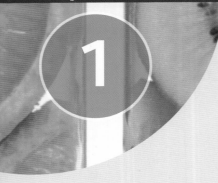

1

In this chapter you have learnt:

✔ that a balanced diet is one which contains all the nutrients we need to keep us healthy

✔ that an unbalanced diet can cause malnutrition

✔ how to use computer programs to carry out nutritional analysis

✔ the function and sources of macronutrients and micronutrients in the diet

✔ how energy is used by the body and the importance of energy balance

✔ about the process of digestion and absorption of nutrients.

Revision quiz

1 Which of the following is the nutrient needed for growth and repair of body cells?

a Protein

b Carbohydrate

c Fat

2 Which of the following nutrients provides the most energy per gram?

a Protein

b Carbohydrate

c Fat

3 Which of the following groups of people have the greatest energy requirement?

a Babies

b Teenagers

c Elderly people

4 Malnutrition is:

a when you eat too much food

b when you don't eat enough food

c when you don't eat the right kinds of foods to meet individual dietary requirements.

5 Males need more energy foods than females because:

a males are more active than females

b males have a higher metabolic rate than females

c males have more body fat than females.

6 Amino acids are found in:

a fats

b vitamins

c proteins.

7 Which of the following foods contains dietary fibre?

a Chicken

b Potatoes

c Cheese

8 Calcium is used in the body to:

a prevent infection

b make red blood cells

c build strong bones and teeth.

9 Which of the following vitamins is an antioxidant?

a Vitamin C

b Vitamin B

c Vitamin D

10 Which of the following foods is a good source of iron in the diet?

a Apples

b Cauliflower

c Red meat

2 Nutritional, physical, chemical and sensory properties of food

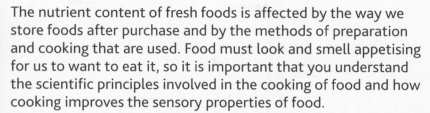

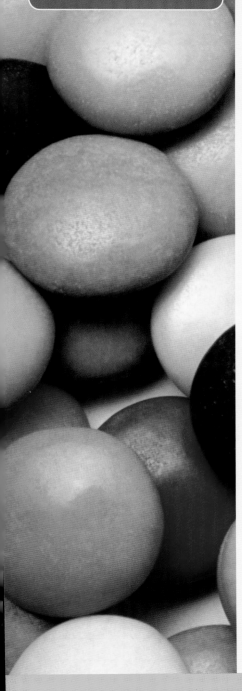

In this chapter:

2.1 Introduction to the effect of storage on nutrients

2.2–2.3 Food preparation and cooking

2.4–2.5 Food additives

The nutrient content of fresh foods is affected by the way we store foods after purchase and by the methods of preparation and cooking that are used. Food must look and smell appetising for us to want to eat it, so it is important that you understand the scientific principles involved in the cooking of food and how cooking improves the sensory properties of food.

Some ready prepared foods contain substances called additives, which are used to make the food safe to eat for longer periods than fresh foods; and to improve the colour, texture or flavour of processed foods.

In this chapter you will learn about:

- the effects of prolonged storage on fats, proteins, carbohydrates and water soluble vitamins
- the loss of vitamin C through oxidation
- the causes of rancidity in fats
- the effect of heat on proteins, fats, sugars, starches and water soluble vitamins
- the loss of water soluble vitamins B and C through soaking, peeling, chopping and cooking
- the scientific principles underlying the cooking of food
- the properties and functions of different ingredients in recipes
- the main functions of food additives in the wider context of food safety, convenience, health and consumer choice
- the use of food additives in product development and to improve nutritional quality
- consumer safeguards for the use of food additives.

What you should already know:

✔ In Chapter 1 you learned about the importance of eating a balanced diet to stay healthy. In this chapter you will learn about the correct methods of storing, preparing and cooking foods in order to get the maximum benefit from the nutritional value of the food.

✔ You may already have some knowledge of additives: in particular colourings which are put into many products aimed at children to make them look appealing.

✔ You may have seen TV investigations on the links between additives and hyperactivity in children.

Introduction to the effect of storage on nutrients

Some nutrients are affected by prolonged storage. In particular, water soluble vitamins B and C are lost as foods lose moisture; and fats can become rancid when stored for long periods.

What are the causes of nutrient loss?

Oxidation

Fresh fruit and vegetables start to lose nutrients as soon as they are harvested. During long periods of storage, and particularly when exposed to oxygen, green vegetables change colour from dark green to yellow and their texture changes from crisp to limp.

Vitamin C, in particular, is lost through oxidation when exposed to oxygen. Air, heat and sunlight speed up the process of oxidation.

Vitamins A and B are also lost when exposed to light.

Rancidity

Fats and oils can develop an unpleasant taste and smell during prolonged storage. This is known as rancidity and is caused by oxidation. Rancidity can affect: hard fats such as butter; vegetable oils; nuts; and foods containing fat such as cakes and biscuits.

Commercially prepared foods often have antioxidants added to prevent fats from becoming rancid and developing an unpleasant taste.

Water loss

Fruit and vegetables begin to lose moisture during storage and dry out, with a loss of the water soluble vitamins B and C.

Enzymes

The action of enzymes can speed up ripening during storage which can change the nutrient content of foods. For example, enzymic action converts starch to sugar in bananas as they ripen.

Enzymes can also cause browning in foods that are cut or bruised, for example apples.

Enzymes (lipases) in fats can cause them to break down into fatty acids.

Objectives

Develop an understanding of the effects of storage time, temperature and exposure to sunlight on the nutrient content of food.

Understand ways in which nutrient losses can be prevented.

Key terms

Oxidation: exposure to air causing loss of vitamin C in fruits and vegetables.

Rancidity: unpleasant flavours which develop in fats when they are exposed to oxygen.

Enzymes: molecules in foods which cause ripening or change the structure.

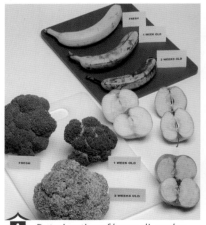

A Deterioration of broccoli, apples and bananas

Practical activity 1

- Carry out a survey of green vegetables from different shops in your area.

- Select one type, such as broccoli or spring cabbage, and compare a sample from a supermarket, greengrocers and corner shop.

- Copy out Table **B** and fill in your results.

B

	Supermarket	Green grocer	Corner shop
Appearance			
Colour			
Smell			
Cost			
Best buy			

Practical activity 2

Working in pairs: cook a small sample of the cabbage or broccoli from each of the shops investigated in practical activity 1, and carry out a sensory analysis of the results.

You will need:

- 3 plates labelled Greengrocer, Corner Shop and Supermarket; samples of broccoli or cabbage bought from each shop; steamer or microwave oven; scales; timer; sharp knife; chopping board.

Method

1. Weigh 50 g of each vegetable sample.

2. Wash each sample well, then cut into medium sized pieces.

3. If microwaving – place the first sample in a small dish, add 1 tablespoon of cold water, cover and cook on high for 4 minutes.

   If steaming – when the water is boiling, place the first sample in the steamer compartment and steam for 8 minutes.

4. Allow to cool before transferring to the appropriately labelled plate.

5. Repeat with second and third samples.

6. Copy out Table **C**, record your results and answer the questions below.

C

	Sample A	Sample B	Sample C
Appearance			
Smell			
Taste			
Texture			
Star rating 1–5			

(See 2.3 and 6.3 for details on star rating.)

7. Which vegetable got the highest star rating?

8. Give reasons why it turned out best.

9. Draw conclusions from your practical work.

Guidelines for preventing nutrient loss

Buying vegetables and fruit

- Buy green vegetables, salads and soft fruits frequently. Use as soon as possible to get the maximum benefit from their vitamin C content.
- Buy local produce and food in season when possible: the storage time before it reaches the shops is shorter. Make sure green vegetables are crisp and bright green with no sign of yellowing

Storage

- Green vegetables should be stored in a cool, dark place – preferably a refrigerator.
- Rancidity in fats can be prevented by storing in a cool, dark place and using before the use by date.

Preparation

Soaking in water, slicing, chopping and grating cause loss of water soluble vitamins B and C, so preparation of green vegetables should be done just before cooking.

Cooking

High temperatures, keeping food warm, and cooking in large amounts of water destroy vitamins B and C. Quick methods of cooking such as stir-frying, microwaving and steaming should be used to conserve these nutrients.

Summary

Nutrients are lost through oxidation, rancidity, and enzymic action.

Fresh foods lose nutrients when stored for long periods.

Food should be eaten as fresh as possible to get the maximum benefit from the nutrients the food provides.

Food preparation and cooking 1

How does preparation and cooking affect the structure and sensory properties of food?

Cooking alters the structure, taste and colour of food in many different ways. For example, boiling potatoes softens their structure and improves the digestibility of the starch content.

The effect of heat on proteins, starches, sugars and fats

Proteins

When protein foods are heated they begin to denature then coagulate at temperatures of around 45 °C to 65 °C for meat, and 60 °C for egg white. **Denaturation** is caused by the breakdown of links in the chains of amino acids which make up protein molecules. If the temperature is raised slowly and kept at around 66 °C the protein will set gradually and will not become too hard.

If the temperature is raised above 100 °C as in frying or roasting, **coagulation** is rapid and the protein hardens where it comes into contact with the heat. High temperatures also cause protein foods to brown, which gives added flavour to the meat and makes the food look more appetising.

Starches

The effect of moist heat on starch is to cause **gelatinisation** to take place, resulting in the food thickening and eventually setting. As the food is heated, the starch grains soften and absorb water. This causes them to swell until they break, making the mixture thicken. This usually takes place at a temperature of 85 °C. If left to go cold, the mixture will become solid.

The effect of dry heat on starch is to cause browning when the starch is turned to dextrin. This is known as **dextrinisation**.

Sugars

The effect of dry heat on sugar is to cause melting, browning or **caramelisation** and, eventually, burning. The effect of moist heat on sugar is to cause the grains to dissolve and, with continued heat, to form a syrup which will caramelise and eventually burn.

Fats

When solid fats are heated they melt at fairly low temperatures. With continued heating, fats will bubble and eventually burn and decompose. 'Smoking point' is reached when fats give off a blue smoke at temperatures of between 130 °C and 200 °C. Oils are liquid at room temperatures but behave in the same way as solid fats, except that their smoking temperature is higher making them more suitable for deep fat frying.

Effect of acid/alkaline conditions on proteins and starches

Proteins

Acids speed up the coagulation processes of proteins in foods such as eggs and milk. In cheese making, an acid starter is added to the milk so

Good examples of protein setting gradually are:

- poached or scrambled eggs

Good examples of protein foods going brown are:

- grilled steak, chops and bacon

Good examples of gelatinisation used in cooking are:

- custards and sauces which use flour or cornflour
- cooking pasta, rice and potatoes

Good examples of dextrinisation in cooking are:

- toasting bread
- browning of cakes, pastries and bread when baking

Good examples of caramelisation are:

- the use of dry heat to brown sugar on top of crème brulée
- the production of spun sugar work for desserts

Key terms

Denaturation: change in chemical structure of proteins during heating.

Coagulation: setting of proteins during heating.

Gelatinisation: thickening of starch when moist heat is applied.

Dextrinisation: browning of starches when dry heat is applied.

Caramelisation: browning of sugar when dry heat is applied.

that the milk proteins begin to set and form solids. Vinegar can be added to the water when poaching eggs, to speed up the setting process.

Acids, such as lemon juice, have a tenderising effect on meat fibres and are often used in marinades.

Starches

Acids and alkalis can be used as raising agents when mixed with starches such as flour. The introduction of acids into set starch can cause the mixture to become runny or curdle.

Practical activity

Investigate the effect of heat on eggs

You will need:

- small mixing bowl, fork, small nonstick pan, wooden spoon, timer, 2 plates, 2 small eggs

Method

1. Crack one egg into bowl and mix well with fork.

2. Start the timer.

3. Pour beaten egg into nonstick pan and cook over a low heat, stirring continuously until mixture begins to thicken.

4. When the egg is set, serve scrambled egg on a plate. Record time taken for the egg to cook.

5. Repeat with second egg, but cook on a high heat.

6. Carry out a sensory analysis of the two methods of making scrambled egg. Comment on your results.

Question

Which sample gave the softest textured scrambled egg and why?

Questions

1. Describe the changes which take place when potatoes are cooked.

2. What is coagulation?

3. What happens to protein foods when they are heated to high temperatures?

4. What is gelatinisation of starch?

5. What is the effect of dry heat on starchy foods?

6. Why is vinegar sometimes added to water used for poaching eggs?

7. What is the smoking point of fat?

8. Why is it dangerous to leave a frying pan containing oil or fat heating unattended on a cooker?

An example of how a mixture can become runny or curdle is:

- the addition of lemon juice to a white sauce

Investigation

Investigate the effects of acids on protein foods

- Pour 50 ml of milk into a measuring jug, stir in 1 tablespoon of vinegar and leave for 10 minutes. What happens to the milk? Why is this?

- Compare boiling or poaching eggs in plain water with water that has had a tablespoon of white vinegar added to it.

Summary

When heated, proteins denature and coagulate.

Moist heat on starch causes gelatinisation.

Dry heat on sugar causes caramelisation.

Food preparation and cooking 2

What are the sensory properties of food?

- Appearance
- Smell
- Taste
- Texture

Effects of preparation and cooking on the sensory properties of food

Appearance and smell

Food has to look and smell appetising to make us want to eat it. The sight and smell of food can start our digestive juices working. Think about walking past a fish and chip shop when you are hungry, or the sight of pastries and cakes in the bakery section of a supermarket.

Retailers use sensory characteristics of food to sell more products: for example, the smell of baking bread in a supermarket.

When we eat food in a café or restaurant we judge it by its initial appearance. Does it look fresh, colourful and attractively served, or tired, limp and kept hot for too long? How the food smells also influences whether we want to eat it, and our sense of smell is very important in protecting us from eating foods which have gone 'off'. Foods which are overcooked or burnt do not look or smell attractive, so we do not want to eat them. Overcooked green vegetables loose their green colour and look yellow or grey, which is unappetising. When we eat out, we want our food to look attractive as well as taste good, and most chefs take time to serve and garnish food so that it is appealing to the customer.

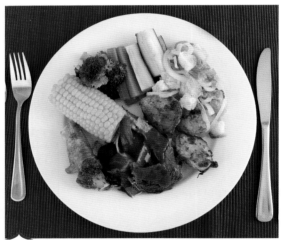

A Food has to look attractive to make us want to eat it

Taste

The taste buds on our tongue detect four basic flavours in food. These are: sweet, sour, salt and savoury. Our personal preferences for food are governed by our taste buds, but are also affected by our sense of smell. Most babies prefer sweet tasting foods, and have to be introduced to savoury flavours through a variety of weaning foods.

Objectives

Understand the effect of preparation and cooking on the sensory properties of food.

Investigation 1

Working in groups of four, brainstorm words which describe the sensory properties of the following foods:

- Pizza
- Chicken curry
- Lemon meringue pie
- Chocolate ice cream

Investigation 2

- Look in food magazines and find pictures of different dishes that you can use to make a colourful chart.
- Add sensory descriptors for each dish to your chart.
- Make a classroom display of your finished charts.

Key terms

Extractives: savoury flavours that develop in meat as it cooks.

Blind tastings: consumer tests on new food products where the tester does not know which food they are tasting.

Cooking alters the taste of many foods: for example, meat develops **extractives**, which give it a savoury flavour; and fat melts and becomes crisp, as with grilled bacon and roast chicken. Cooking also improves the taste and digestibility of starchy foods such as potatoes.

Texture

A variety of textures from different foods improves our enjoyment of a meal. Textures can be described as: crisp, crunchy, chewy, smooth, greasy, runny, dry, hard, soft etc. Ideally, a meal should contain some crunchy or chewy foods with some smooth or soft foods: for example, sausages and mash; beans on toast; or apple pie and custard.

Cooking affects the texture of foods by: softening, for example boiling potatoes or vegetables; tenderising, for example roasting or stewing meat; making the food crisp, as in deep frying, toasting or baking.

Sensory analysis

This is a process carried out to analyse a food product using our senses of sight, smell, taste and hearing. It is usually carried out with a group of consumers who test new products for food manufacturers. Testings are usually 'blind tastings', where the taster does not know the identity of each product tested. The words used to describe these tastings are known as sensory descriptors.

Rules for carrying out taste tests

1   Use at least four people to test the food, and do not allow them to discuss the results with each other.
2   Provide glasses of water for them to sip in order to clear their palates in between each tasting.
3   Serve the food samples on identical plates or dishes. Label each one A, B, C, D etc. so you can indentify them later.
4   Before they start, inform the tasters how to taste each sample and fill in the table. Provide them with a word bank of sensory descriptors.
5   Record the results of the taste tests using one or more of the methods opposite.

Computer spreadsheet programs can be used to present your results as charts or graphs for all of the methods shown.

B   Table with comments

	Food A	Food B
Appearance		
Taste		
Texture		
Smell		
Overall score 1–5		

C   Ranking test: where foods are ranked in order of preference

Food	Order	Comments
A		
B		
C		
D		

D   Rating test: where foods are given a score, usually from 1–5

	Food A	Food B
1. Did not like at all		
2. Disliked slightly		
3. No preference		
4. Liked a little		
5. Liked a lot		

E   Star Profile
This is a good method of presenting the results of a ranking or rating test. Different colours can be used for each person on the tasting panel so that comparisons can be made of the results. (See 6.3 for an example.)

Summary

Cooking affects the colour, flavour and texture of food.

Without cooking some foods, such as potatoes, would be unpalatable.

Sensory properties of food include appearance, colour, flavour, texture and smell.

2.4 Food additives 1

What are food additives?

Processed foods often contain very small amounts of ingredients which are added to extend their shelf life, or to improve their colour, texture, flavour or nutritional value. **Food additives** can be from natural or synthetic (chemical) sources. Examples of natural additives are salt, and acids such as vinegar and lemon juice. Examples of synthetic additives are saccharin and aspartame sweeteners.

Why are additives used?

- To improve the shelf life of the product: that is the length of time the food is safe to eat.
- To improve the flavour, texture, appearance, colour or smell of the food.
- To improve the consistency of food.
- To increase nutritional value.

Types of additives and their uses

Preservatives

These are used to prevent decay and make food safe to eat for longer periods. Used in bacon, sausages, cooked meats and pies.

Antioxidants

These are used to prevent fats and oils from becoming rancid. Used in most products which include fat, such as cakes, biscuits and pastries.

Colourings

As their name suggests, these are used to add colour to products such as sweets, yogurts, desserts, tinned peas and soups.

Flavourings

These are used to add flavour to products such as ice cream, chocolate mousse, yogurts, crisps and soft drinks.

Flavour enhancers

Flavour enhancers, such as monosodium glutamate, are used to give a more intense flavour to foods such as meat, ready meals and cook-in sauces. Sweeteners, such as saccharin, give a sweeter flavour than sugar and can be used in 'sugar free' products.

Emulsifiers

Used to mix water and oil together in a stable solution and to prevent separation. They are used in products such as salad dressings, mayonnaise and low fat spreads.

Stabilisers

These are similar to emulsifiers and are used to prevent separation. Used in many products, but good examples are cook-in sauces and yogurts.

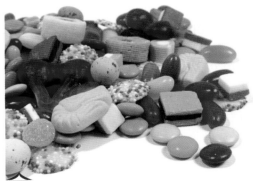

A Colourings are used to make foods look attractive

Nutritional supplements

These are added to enrich foods: for example, vitamins A and D are added to margarine; calcium is added by law to white bread, which is also fortified with iron, thiamin and nicotinic acid; iron is added to some cereals; and vitamin C is added to fruit juice and many other products.

Should we worry about food additives?

All additives that are **permitted** for use by food manufacturers in the UK have been rigorously tested to make sure they are safe to eat. Once they have been tested, they are registered and given an **E number**, which means they can be used in countries in the European Union. For example, E412 is a stabiliser called guargum which is often used in desserts.

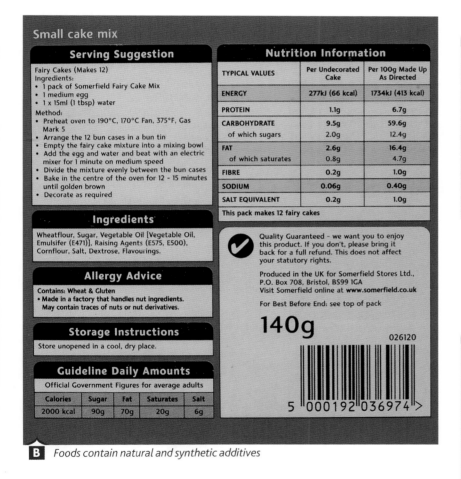

B   *Foods contain natural and synthetic additives*

Key terms

Food additive: natural or chemical substance added to food to improve quality.

Permitted additives: tested by the Food Standards Agency before being approved for use by food manufacturers.

E numbers: additives approved by the European Union.

Investigation

Look at the label shown in Photo **B** and answer the following questions.

1. Which of the ingredients listed are natural additives and which are synthetic additives?

2. What are the functions of each additive?

Questions

1. What are permitted additives?

2. What does the 'E' in E number mean?

3. Describe how food additives give the consumer greater choice when shopping for food.

Summary

Additives can be natural or synthetic.

Permitted additives are given an E number.

Without additives, we would not have such a wide range of foods available to us.

Use of additives to improve nutritional quality of food

Food manufacturers have added nutrients to some foods for many years. These foods include: breakfast cereals, which are **fortified** with vitamins and minerals; white flour and bread, which have calcium, iron and B vitamins added; and margarine which has vitamins A and D added by law.

Fruit juices and children's drinks often have added vitamin C, and sports drinks have added minerals and glucose to replace nutrients lost during exercise.

Novel foods

Quorn is a **novel food** made from myco-protein which was developed by RHM in the late 1960s. Quorn is low in fat and high in protein.

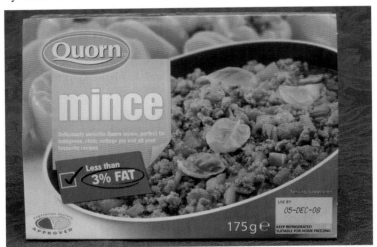

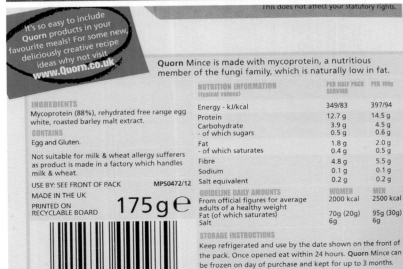

Quorn Mince is made with mycoprotein, a nutritious member of the fungi family, which is naturally low in fat.

INGREDIENTS
Mycoprotein (88%), rehydrated free range egg white, roasted barley malt extract.

CONTAINS
Egg and Gluten.

Not suitable for milk & wheat allergy sufferers as product is made in a factory which handles milk & wheat.

USE BY: SEE FRONT OF PACK   MPS0472/12
MADE IN THE UK
PRINTED ON
RECYCLABLE BOARD   **175g℮**

NUTRITION INFORMATION (typical values)	PER HALF PACK SERVING	PER 100g
Energy - kJ/kcal	349/83	397/94
Protein	12.7 g	14.5 g
Carbohydrate	3.9 g	4.5 g
- of which sugars	0.5 g	0.6 g
Fat	1.8 g	2.0 g
- of which saturates	0.4 g	0.5 g
Fibre	4.8 g	5.5 g
Sodium	0.1 g	0.1 g
Salt equivalent	0.2 g	0.2 g

GUIDELINE DAILY AMOUNTS From official figures for average adults of a healthy weight	WOMEN 2000 kcal	MEN 2500 kcal
Fat (of which saturates)	70g (20g)	95g (30g)
Salt	6g	6g

STORAGE INSTRUCTIONS
Keep refrigerated and use by the date shown on the front of the pack. Once opened eat within 24 hours. **Quorn** Mince can be frozen on day of purchase and kept for up to 3 months. **Do not refreeze once thawed.**

Quorn™ and the **Quorn™** logo are trademarks of Marlow Foods Ltd.

5 019503 000979

B *Quorn™ is a novel food*

Practical activity

- Make a main meal for four students using Quorn™ mince instead of meat mince: spaghetti bolognese, for example.
- Carry out a sensory analysis of the finished dish, and record your comments in a table.
- Work out the nutrient content of one portion of the spaghetti bolognese and compare it with the same recipe made with meat.
- Evaluate your results.

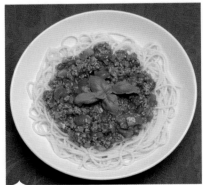

A *Spaghetti bolognese made with Quorn™*

Investigation

- Look at Photo **B** and compare the protein, fat and fibre content of 100g Quorn chunks with 100g chicken.

Are there any advantages of food additives?

- Without additives we would not have such a wide variety of food available in the form of pre-prepared and processed food. For example, breakfast cereals are one of the most popular processed foods in this country and are eaten by most people every day. If you look on a cereal packet you will see that most contain some additives as well as vitamin and mineral fortification.
- Foods such as yogurts and ice cream would separate and go runny without stabilisers and emulsifiers, and cakes and biscuits would taste stale without antioxidants.
- Preservatives make food safe to eat for longer periods and prevent mould growth on some foods.
- Colourings make foods such as jellies, sweets and desserts look more appetising. Tinned fruits and vegetables would look grey without colourings. Many colourings are now made from natural ingredients such as fruit juices and caramelised sugar.
- Some additives increase the nutritional value of foods, for example vitamins added to cereals and bread.
- Additives enable consumers to store foods for longer periods, which means that shopping for food can be done when it is convenient.

Are there any disadvantages of food additives?

There is growing concern, particularly among some parents, that additives may cause allergies and hyperactivity in children. Food colourings are mainly blamed, so many manufacturers of foods aimed at children claim that their products are additive free. Providing plenty of fresh foods are eaten, a small amount of foods containing permitted additives can be included in a healthy diet.

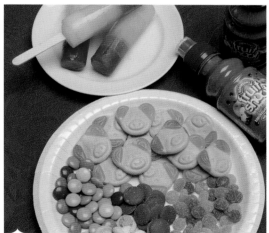

C   *Children's sweets and drinks which are advertised as additive free*

Summary

Additives are used to improve the nutritional quality of food.

Additives such as preservatives prevent foods deteriorating and causing food poisoning.

Some parents are concerned that additives may cause hyperactivity in children.

Key terms

Fortified: where nutrients are added to improve the nutritional value of a product.

Novel foods: foods which are manufactured from ingredients not normally used for food.

Appetising: looks and smells good to eat.

AQA   Examiner's tip

Be able to describe the advantages and disadvantages of the use of food additives.

Questions

1.   Give **three** examples of foods which are fortified with vitamins and minerals?

2.   Which nutrients are added to white flour and bread?

3.   Which vitamins are added to margarine by law?

4.   What is the purpose of added minerals in sports drinks?

5.   What is Quorn?

6.   Give **three** examples of the advantages of food additives.

7.   What are the disadvantages of food additives?

8.   Suggest how foods containing additives can be included in a healthy diet.

2

In this chapter you have learnt:

✔ the effect of prolonged storage on the nutritional value of foods

✔ that water soluble vitamins B and C are lost when fresh fruit and vegetables are stored, prepared and cooked

✔ how the application of heat affects proteins, starches, sugars and fats

✔ how acids and alkalis affect proteins and starches

✔ that cooking alters the sensory properties (appearance, smell, taste and texture) of food

✔ about the function and safe use of food additives in product development.

Revision quiz

1 When green vegetables are exposed to sunlight, vitamin C is lost through:

a rancidity

b oxidation

c enzymic action.

2 Which of the following will be the best source of vitamin C?

a Spring cabbage which has just been boiled with bicarbonate of soda

b Spring cabbage which has been steamed for 10 minutes

c Spring cabbage which has been microwaved for 4 minutes

3 Loss of water soluble vitamins B and C is caused by:

a soaking in water

b slicing, grating and chopping

c all of these.

4 Denaturation of proteins is caused by:

a heating

b storage

c freezing.

5 Gelatinisation of starches causes the mixture to:

a look shiny

b thicken

c brown.

6 Dextrinisation is caused by:

a moist heat on sugar

b moist heat on starch

c dry heat on starch.

7 When ranking tests are carried out, food tasters are asked to:

a make comments on the food tasted

b put the foods in order of preference

c use a star profile to record their results.

8 Which of the following is a natural additive?

a Saccharin

b E412

c Salt

9 Permitted additives are given an E number. This means:

a they have been tested to make sure they are safe to eat

b they have been tested, registered and can be used in all the countries in the European Union

c they contain emulsifiers.

10 Some people are concerned that food additives might cause:

a hyperactivity

b obesity

c diabetes.

3

Techniques and skills in food storage, preparation and cooking

In this chapter:

3.1 Food storage

3.2–3.3 Food preparation and cooking

3.4–3.5 Cooking methods

3.6 Recipe balance and modification

3.7 Convenience foods

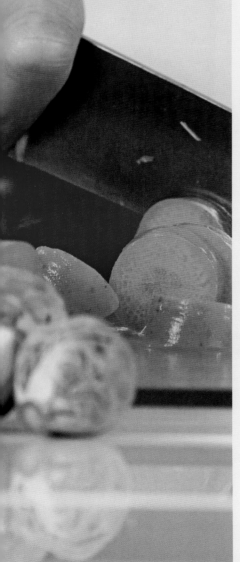

Many people will shop for food once a week in a large supermarket. They will buy a wide variety of perishable (fresh) and non-perishable foods (dry goods), which must be stored correctly until the food is eaten. For example, fresh produce such as meat, dairy products and vegetables must be stored in a fridge and frozen foods must be stored in a freezer. Dry goods which are packed in tins, jars and packets can be stored in cupboards and larders.

In this chapter you will learn about:

- the importance of storing foods correctly to prevent food poisoning
- the avoidance of cross-contamination between raw and cooked foods
- organisational and management skills required for the preparation and cooking of food
- the function of small and large kitchen equipment
- the different types of time, energy and labour saving kitchen equipment
- the different reasons for cooking food
- the methods of heat transfer involved in different methods of cooking food
- the function of ingredients in: sweetening, browning, aeration, enriching, shortening, flavouring and adding structure to recipes
- the effect of combining ingredients in a wide variety of food preparation and cooking
- modification of recipes to reduce the fat, salt and sugar content and to increase dietary fibre
- the application of nutritional guidelines to existing recipes.

■ What you should already know:

✔ In Chapter 2 you learned about the effect of storage on the nutritional value of some nutrients and the ways in which prolonged storage can affect the sensory properties of food.

✔ You also learned about the scientific principles involved in the preparation and cooking of food which you will need to consider when you modify recipes to make them healthier.

3.1 Food storage

Why must food be stored correctly?

Food must be stored correctly to maintain its freshness, palatability and to ensure it is safe to eat.

Objectives

Understand the importance of storing foods correctly.

Types of foods

Foods can be grouped into two types: **perishable** (fresh foods) and **non-perishable** (dry goods).

Perishable foods

Fresh foods need to be stored in a refrigerator at temperatures of 1–5 °C as soon as they are bought, otherwise they will very soon become unfit to eat. They need to be wrapped to exclude air and to prevent tainting with flavours from other foods. Suitable packaging for storing foods in a fridge includes foil, plastic film, and plastic boxes with tightly fitting lids.

Some fresh foods such as meat and bread can be stored in the freezer. Foods which are frozen must be well packaged with foil, plastic bags or plastic film specially made for freezing, to prevent the food from drying out.

A *Storage of perishable foods*

Perishable food	Storage in fridge	Safe storage time
Raw meat, chicken and fish	Bottom shelf, well away from cooked foods.	1–2 days, or until use by date.
Milk, eggs	Bottle rack, egg rack (or in egg box).	Until use by date.
Butter, margarine, yogurts	Top shelf.	Until use by date.
Cooked meats, paté, cheese, desserts	Middle shelf.	Until use by date.
Vegetables and salads	Salad drawer.	2–3 days, or until use by date.

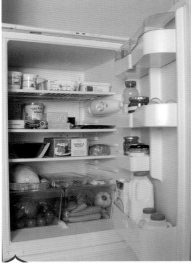

B *How fresh foods should be stored in a fridge*

Non-perishable foods

These foods have been processed in some way and are usually stored in cupboards. They include foods in tins, packets, jars and vacuum packs. All these foods carry a date mark to advise the consumer on the period of time when the food is safe to eat. Store cupboards should be kept clean and airy to prevent infestation from pests. Date marks should be checked frequently so that the oldest food is used first: this is known as stock rotation.

C *Storage of non-perishable foods*

Non-perishable food	Storage	Safe storage time
Flour, pasta, rice, sugar	Dry cupboard in sealed containers.	Up to 1 year or until best before date.
Tinned foods	Dry cupboard.	Until best before date.
Breakfast cereals, tea, coffee	Sealed containers or tins.	Until best before date.
Herbs and spices	Away from sunlight in dry cupboard.	3–4 months.
Bread	Sealed plastic bags, or bread bins.	2–3 days, or until best before date.

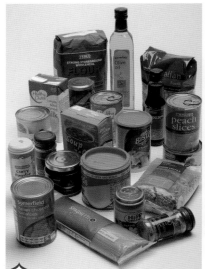

D *A selection of non-perishable foods*

Practical activity

Comparison of different types of packaging materials

Working in pairs you will need:

- 1 cooking apple or 100 g broccoli
- large pan of boiling water
- bowl of ice cold water
- timer, colander and sieve
- packaging materials and containers such as: foil, cling film, plastic bags (ordinary and freezer bags) and plastic boxes with tightly fitting lids
- drinking straw and freezer labels.

Method

1. Peel and slice apple or cut broccoli into florets.
2. When water in pan is boiling, drop in apple slices or broccoli and **blanch** for 2 minutes.
3. Drain off boiling water and plunge apple slices or broccoli into iced water for 2 minutes.
4. Drain and allow to go cold.
5. Choose suitable packaging material for the apple or broccoli and pack, excluding as much air as possible. (Drinking straws can be used to remove air from plastic bags.)
6. Seal and label and place in the freezer for at least 3 weeks.
7. Remove the apple and broccoli samples from the freezer and allow to thaw out.
8. Observe the colour and texture of the samples and any deterioration which has taken place.
9. Note which packaging material was most successful in preserving the freshness of the broccoli and apples.
10. Record your results in a table.

Questions

1. Why must food be stored correctly?
2. What is the difference between perishable and non-perishable foods?
3. Why must foods be wrapped before storing in the fridge or freezer?
4. What are suitable wrapping materials for food stored in a freezer?
5. What are the storage instructions for the following foods: fresh lamb chops, tomatoes, dried pasta, a loaf of sliced bread?
6. What is stock rotation?

Key terms

Perishable: fresh foods which decay rapidly.

Non-perishable: foods which have been processed to prevent rapid decay.

Blanch: cooking vegetables or fruit in boiling water for short periods to inactivate enzymes which may cause deterioration.

AQA Examiner's tip

Make sure you know how to store fresh foods correctly in the fridge.

Remember

Foods which are frozen must be packaged in plastic bags or containers suitable for freezing, with as much air as possible excluded.

Summary

Perishable foods are fresh foods which need to be stored in the fridge.

Non-perishable foods, also known as dry goods, have been processed to extend their shelf life.

Stock rotation is using the oldest food first.

■ Why are organisational and management skills important when preparing and cooking food?

Whether you are a celebrity chef cooking meals at a top restaurant or a parent making meals for a family, you have to be organised in the kitchen to make sure your meals are appetising and ready on time.

To cook meals successfully you need:

- to **organise** your resources: for example, equipment and ingredients.
- to manage your time: for example, shopping time to buy the ingredients; preparation and cooking time; and washing up and clearing away time.
- to develop your practical cookery skills so that you can make a wide range of different dishes.
- to be able to use a range of large and small kitchen equipment safely and **efficiently**.
- to understand the rules of kitchen hygiene and safety.

Objectives

Develop the ability to organise time and effort.

Be able to select and use a range of small kitchen equipment competently.

Key terms

Organised: using good working practice.

Efficient: performing a task without wasting time and energy.

Remember

Be well organised and hygienic in the kitchen if you want your practical work to be successful.

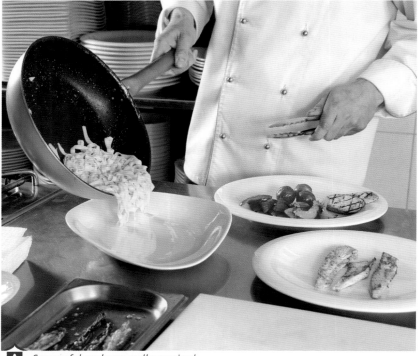

A   *Successful cooks are well organised*

■ Selecting kitchen equipment

There is a wide range of small and large kitchen equipment available in the shops, and it is very tempting to buy things you may not use very much. Equipping a kitchen need not be expensive if you stick to buying equipment that you will use most days. Kitchen equipment is made up of: knives, wooden spoons and other utensils; bowls and pans; and pieces of electrical equipment which save time and effort.

AQA Examiner's tip

Next time you are in a large department store, look at the range of small kitchen equipment available and assess its usefulness.

Small equipment should include:

Chopping boards

These can be made of wood, plastic or toughened glass. Plastic ones are available in different colours so that one can be kept for raw meat only. This helps to avoid cross-contamination with other foods.

Kitchen scales

A good set of scales is necessary for accurate weighing of ingredients. Scales come in many different designs but the basic types are: balances, which use weights; spring balances, which have a dial and usually a scale pan on top; and electronic scales, which need batteries to operate them. The choice of weighing scales depends on the personal preference of the cook.

Kitchen knives

A selection of large and small kitchen knives are needed for different purposes. For example, a large cook's knife for chopping; a bread knife with a serrated edge to make slicing bread easier; and a small knife for vegetable preparation. Kitchen knives can be bought as a set of different sizes in a storage block.

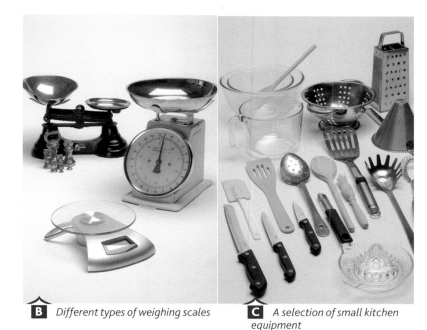

B *Different types of weighing scales*

C *A selection of small kitchen equipment*

Investigation

- Compare peeling apples or carrots with: a vegetable peeler; a small vegetable knife; a table knife. Weigh the peelings from each and comment on your results.
- A young couple who like cooking are buying kitchen equipment for a new flat. Give advice on the small equipment they should buy and the reasons why it is needed.

Other small equipment includes:

mixing bowls, wooden spoons, measuring jugs, sieves, colanders, spatulas, graters, baking trays and cake tins.

Summary

Successful cooks organise resources such as equipment and ingredients effectively.

Small kitchen equipment should be selected carefully, so that money is not wasted on unused utensils.

Questions

1 What are the skills needed by the cook to be able to produce meals successfully?

2 Which type of chopping board would you use for cutting up raw meat?

3 What are the different types of kitchen scales?

Electrical equipment should include:

Microwave ovens

- Save time: food cooks very quickly cutting cooking times by up to 75 per cent.
- Save money: because food cooks more quickly, microwave cooking uses less power and is therefore cheaper than using a conventional oven.
- Save washing up: because dishes can be used for both cooking and serving.
- Can be used for thawing frozen foods, cooking and reheating.
- Are easier to clean than a conventional cooker.
- Are safe to use, as they do not get hot on the outside.
- Are available in different categories from A to E, based on the power output measured in watts. The higher the wattage the faster the food cooks.

Food processors

- Save time when chopping, slicing and puréeing vegetables.
- Can be used for flour mixtures, such as blending and rubbing in, or for making bread dough.
- Can be used for grating cheese and making breadcrumbs.
- Can be used for grinding nuts and spices.
- Goblet and blade can be washed in a dishwasher.

Blenders (sometimes called liquidisers)

- Come in two types, goblet and hand-held.
- Goblet types have similar uses to food processors, but are particularly good for making fruit purées and smoothies.
- Hand-held blenders are more convenient to use for blending soups and baby foods.

Food mixers

- Can be hand-held models or free-standing with a bowl and a stand.
- Hand-held mixers are useful for whipping cream and whisking egg whites. They are easily cleaned and stored.
- Free-standing mixers are more powerful than hand-held and have a variety of different attachments. For example, dough hooks for making bread dough; beaters for making cake mixtures; and whisks for making large quantities of whisked egg mixture.
- Some also have mincers and sausage making attachments. These food mixers are expensive, so they should only be bought if they will be used regularly.

Objectives

Understand the importance of safe and hygienic use of kitchen equipment during preparation and cooking of food.

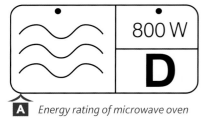

A *Energy rating of microwave oven*

Practical activity 1

Compare the cooking time, cost of energy, appearance, texture and taste of jacket potatoes cooked in a microwave, with those cooked in a conventional oven.

Practical activity 2

- Compare and contrast shortcrust pastry made by hand, with that made in a food processor.
- Use the pastry to make a fruit pie or a cheese and onion quiche.

Remember

You can save time and effort in food preparation and cooking by using electrical kitchen equipment.

Safe, effective and hygienic use of kitchen equipment

Non-electrical equipment

- Always use a chopping board when chopping with sharp knives.
- Do not leave sharp knives soaking in a bowl of washing up water: someone may put their hand in and cut their fingers. Always wash and dry sharp knives carefully and put them away.
- Wash all small equipment in hot soapy water, rinse and dry before putting away.
- Most bowls, pans and cookware can be washed in a dishwasher.
- Products made from wood are not suitable for washing in dishwashers.

Small electrical equipment

- Do not run food processors, blenders or mixers for longer than is necessary, as this may cause the motor to overheat and wear out.
- Do not overfill the bowl or goblet, as this can be dangerous with hot liquids such as soup.
- Keep electrical plugs and sockets away from water and do not plug in electrical equipment with wet hands, as you can get an electric shock.
- Take care when using hand-held blenders and whisks. Only switch them on when they are held down inside the pan or bowl, and switch off before removing them.
- Wash bowl or goblet, beaters, blades and other attachments in hot soapy water after use and take care when handling blades or slicing plates.

Microwave ovens

- Wipe out with a damp clean cloth after each use.
- Periodically, or after cooking strongly flavoured foods, wash out the inside of the microwave with hot soapy water, rinse and dry.

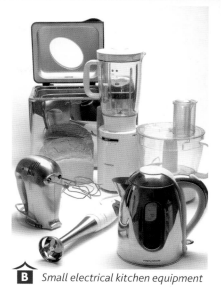

B *Small electrical kitchen equipment*

Key terms

Energy saving: using less power, such as electricity or gas.

Labour saving: saving effort by the cook.

Investigation

- Working in groups, select one piece of electrical equipment and investigate: the types available; features; uses; power rating; and costs.
- Prepare a consumer style report on your research.
- Carry out some practical tests to assess the time, **energy** and **labour saving** features.

Questions

1. List **five** advantages of cooking in a microwave oven.
2. Give **three** examples of ways in which food processors can save time.
3. Which piece of electrical equipment could be used for each of the following?
   a. Making breadcrumbs
   b. Making a fruit smoothie
   c. Blending soup
4. List **four** safety rules that must be observed when using electrical equipment.

Summary

Microwave ovens save time and electricity compared with conventional ovens.

Food processors save time and effort when slicing and puréeing vegetables.

All kitchen equipment should be kept clean and grease free, to prevent contamination of food.

Care should be taken when using electrical equipment and sharp blades.

What are the reasons for cooking foods?

- To kill bacteria and make food such as raw meat and eggs safe to eat.
- To develop flavours and improve the taste (**organoleptic** characteristics) of food.
- To soften fibres in meat and vegetables and make them easier to eat and digest.
- To improve the keeping qualities of foods so that they can be used for longer periods.
- To give variety to the diet.

Heat transfer

Heat transfer is the process by which heat energy is transferred to the food from the cooker. There are many different ways of cooking food, but they all use one of three methods of heat transfer, which are: **convection**, **conduction** and **radiation**.

Convection

Heat moves through liquids and gases by convection currents. For example, when boiling vegetables in a pan of water, the water expands and rises as it is heated and cooler water takes its place at the base of the pan; the cooler water is in turn heated until all the water reaches boiling point. Ovens are also heated by convection currents: the hot air rises making the oven hotter at the top and cooler at the bottom, producing different **zones of heat**.

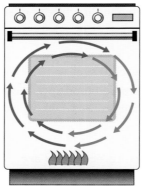

A *Convection currents in an oven*

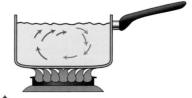

B *Convection currents in a sauce-pan of water*

Conduction

Heat is conducted through molecules in solids or liquids. When a metal saucepan is placed on the heat source it heats up because the molecules in the metal start to vibrate. If the pan is filled with water the molecules in the water vibrate faster and heat up. Metals and water are good conductors of heat, but wood, plastic and cotton are poor conductors of heat.

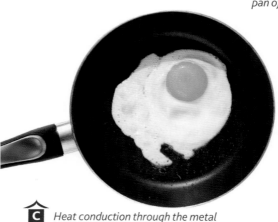

C *Heat conduction through the metal base of a frying pan*

Radiation

Heating by radiation takes place when heat is transferred directly onto food by infra-red rays from the heat source. Good examples of cooking by radiation are toasting bread in a toaster and cooking sausages under a grill.

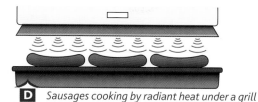

D *Sausages cooking by radiant heat under a grill*

Microwaves

Microwave ovens use electromagnetic waves to cook food. The magnetron in the oven generates microwave energy, which penetrates the water molecules in the food, causing them to vibrate and give off heat. The food becomes hot, but the oven itself stays cool. Microwaves are a form of radiation.

Practical activity

Experimental work on heat transfer

Working in groups:

1 Preheat a convection oven (not a fan oven) to 190 °C.

2 Make up a 200 g batch of scone mixture and cut into 9 small scones all of the same thickness.

3 Place 3 scones on each of 3 baking trays.

4 Cook the first tray on the top shelf, the second tray on the middle shelf, and the third tray on the bottom shelf.

5 Bake the scones for 15 minutes.

6 When the time is up, remove all three trays from the oven.

7 Measure the height of the scones and observe their colour, taste and texture.

8 Copy Table **E**, and record your observations.

E

Scone batches	Height	Colour	Texture	Taste
Cooked on top shelf				
Cooked on middle shelf				
Cooked on bottom shelf				

3.5 Cooking methods 2

Objectives

Understand the advantages and disadvantages of moist and dry methods of cooking.

Methods of cooking

A *Methods of cooking*

Moist methods	Method of heat transfer	Suitable foods	Advantages	Disadvantages
Boiling (water reaches 100 °C)	Conduction through pan and convection through water.	Eggs, pasta, rice, potatoes, vegetables	• Quick method, used for many foods. • Economical use of fuel.	• Water soluble nutrients lost. • Flavour lost from meat. • Overcooking causes some food to disintegrate, e.g. pasta and potatoes.
Poaching (water kept at 63 °C)	Conduction through pan and convection through water.	Fish, chicken, eggs, fruit	• Gentle method of cooking. • Does not cause food to break up.	• Some loss of water soluble nutrients. • Food may be bland and require flavouring ingredients added to the water.
Steaming	Convection and conduction.	Vegetables, puddings, fish	• Food does not come into direct contact with the water, so less loss of water soluble vitamins.	• Some foods take a long time to cook in a steamer. • Can cause a great deal of condensation in the kitchen.
Stewing	Conduction through dish and convection through liquid.	Meat, vegetables, fruit	• Tenderises tough cuts of meat, as it is a long slow method of cooking. • Nutrient loss is kept to the minimum, as the liquid is served with the food.	• Takes a long time to cook, so meal has to be planned well in advance. • Uneconomical to heat oven for long periods to cook one dish.
Pressure cooking	Conduction through pan and convection through water.	Meat, vegetables	• Fast method of cooking. • Economical use of fuel.	• Food tends to lose texture and can taste bland.
Dry methods				
Roasting	Convection and conduction through roasting tin.	Meat, chicken, vegetables	• Tenderises joints of meat. • Develops extractives, giving more flavour. • Little attention needed during cooking. • Vegetables can be roasted with the meat.	• Food dries out and proteins can toughen at high cooking temperatures. • Fat splashes from roasting can cause a greasy oven.
Baking	Convection and conduction through baking tin.	Flour mixtures, potatoes, apples, vegetables, fish	• Gives attractive appearance and flavour. • Several items can be cooked in the oven at once.	• Flour mixtures need constant attention during cooking. • Some mixtures with large amounts of sugar burn easily.
Grilling	Radiation.	Meat, including sausages and bacon; cheese on toast; fish	• Quick method of cooking, suitable for snacks.	• Requires constant attention as food easily burns.
Frying methods				
Deep frying	Conduction through the pan and convection through the fat.	Chips, fish, scotch eggs, fritters, chicken	• Quick method. • Suitable for many types of foods.	• Food absorbs large amounts of fat, which is not very healthy. • Chip pans on cookers are very dangerous, and need constant attention.
Shallow frying	Conduction through the pan and convection through the fat.	Sausages, eggs, tomatoes, fish fingers	• Quick method. • Suitable for many types of food.	• Uses less fat than deep frying, but food still absorbs fat.
Stir-frying	Conduction through the pan and convection through the food.	Vegetables, chicken, noodles	Healthy as: • small amount of oil used • food is cooked quickly, minimising nutrient loss.	• Needs constant attention to avoid over cooking.

Methods of cooking vegetables to reduce nutrient loss

As we found out in Chapter 2, cooking alters the flavour of foods and may destroy some vitamins in vegetables. Some cooking methods are better than others for conserving the nutrient value, flavour and texture of vegetables. These are usually quick methods of cooking at high temperatures using very small amounts of water or oil. Steaming and cooking vegetables in a microwave are good methods for conserving water soluble vitamins B and C, as the vegetables do not come into contact with water. Stir-frying vegetables also conserves nutrients, as this is a quick method of cooking which uses a very small amount of oil.

Guidelines for cooking vegetables to reduce nutrient loss

- Make sure vegetables are as fresh as possible.
- Cut them into small sections (or shred cabbage finely) just before cooking.
- For boiling – cover the base of the saucepan with 1 cm of water and bring to a rapid boil before adding vegetables. Cover pan with a tightly fitting lid and boil rapidly for 6 minutes. Check whilst cooking that the pan does not boil dry. Strain vegetables and use any liquid left in gravy or stock, as it contains water soluble vitamins.
- For steaming – bring the water to the boil in the steamer then add the vegetables to the steaming compartment and cover with a lid. Steam for 6 minutes, drain and serve.
- For microwaving – place prepared vegetables in a microwavable dish; add a small amount of water; cover with clingfilm and microwave on high for 4 minutes.

Remember

Moist methods of cooking and high temperatures destroy water soluble vitamins B and C. To conserve these vitamins in vegetables, steam, microwave or stir-fry them.

Key terms

Moist methods: cooking with added liquid.

Dry methods: cooking with no added liquid, but fat sometimes used to prevent food sticking to tins.

AQA Examiner's tip

Next time you have a practical cookery lesson, make a note of the different cooking methods you use.

Practical activity

Working in groups:
- prepare and cook a selection of seasonal vegetables using as many different cooking methods as possible.
- prepare a class display of the finished results and produce a table to record your comments.

B

Vegetable	Method of cooking	Cooking time	Appearance	Taste	Texture	Score out of 10

Summary

The choice of method of cooking depends on the time available and the food to be cooked.

Each different method of cooking has advantages and disadvantages.

Conservative method of cooking – quick method using a small amount of water or oil to conserve nutrients.

Questions

Look at the information in Table **A** and answer the following questions.

1 What are the advantages and disadvantages of stewing and pressure cooking?

2 Compare and contrast boiling and steaming as methods of cooking.

3 What are the advantages and disadvantages of roasting and grilling?

4 Compare and contrast shallow frying and stir-frying.

3.6 Recipe balance and modification

What is recipe balance?

Recipe balance is the combination of ingredients that gives a successful end product. In order to **modify** or change recipes, it is important to understand the function of ingredients in recipes.

Function of ingredients in recipes

Sweetness – Sugar; honey; fruit purées such as apple, apricot or pear; dried fruits; and fresh fruits such as bananas.

Browning – Meat juices when cooked; caramelised sugar; egg glaze.

Flavouring – In savoury dishes: salt and pepper, herbs and spices, garlic, tomato purée, mustard and soy sauce. In sweet dishes: chocolate, coffee, nuts, vanilla, lemon, strawberry and raspberry.

Emulsifying – Lecithin in egg yolk acts as an emulsifying agent, in mayonnaise for example, and helps to hold oil and water in suspension.

Aeration – Flour mixtures are made lighter by adding air, gas or steam. Air is added through sieving flour, whisking eggs, creaming fat and sugar, and beating batters. Gas, in the form of carbon dioxide, is produced from raising agents such as yeast in bread, and baking powder in cakes. Steam is produced when mixtures with a large amount of liquid in them are cooked at high temperatures: for example, batters made into Yorkshire puddings.

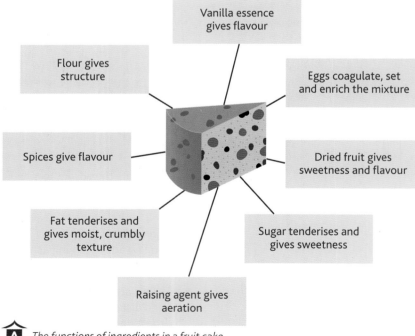

Vanilla essence gives flavour

Flour gives structure

Spices give flavour

Fat tenderises and gives moist, crumbly texture

Raising agent gives aeration

Eggs coagulate, set and enrich the mixture

Dried fruit gives sweetness and flavour

Sugar tenderises and gives sweetness

A *The functions of ingredients in a fruit cake*

Structure – Flour mixtures containing raising agents will rise in the oven because the raising agents produce air, gas and steam which all expand when heated. As they expand, they push up the flour mixture until the proteins in the flour harden and set the structure in the risen shape. If the mixture also contains eggs, the protein in the eggs coagulates and helps to give a firmer structure.

Tenderising – Fats and oils shorten, or tenderise, flour mixtures giving a moist, melt in the mouth texture. The more fat a recipe contains the richer and moister the finished product. For example, creaming method cakes have equal quantities of fat to flour. High proportions of sugar in baked goods also give a finer crumb and softer texture.

Enriching – Butter, cream, egg yolks and cheese can be added to enrich mixtures.

Preserving – Salt and vinegar are used in pickling; and sugar is used in jam making.

B *Methods of aeration used in baked flour products*

Product	Method of aeration	Type of flour
Bread	Carbon dioxide from yeast.	Plain
Batters	Steam from liquid content of recipe.	Plain
Whisked sponge cakes and swiss roll	Air from sieving flour and whisking eggs.	Plain
Victoria sandwich cake; biscuits and scones	Air from sieving flour and creaming margarine and sugar. Carbon dioxide from baking powder.	Self-raising
Pastry	Air from sieving flour, rubbing in, and folding and rolling.	Plain

Practical activity

Modifying recipes

- Make spaghetti bolognese using flavouring ingredients instead of salt. Using a nutritional analysis program, compare the salt content of your home made version with a jar of bolognese sauce.

- Working in pairs, make a batch of traditional all-in-one method buns and a batch of all-in-one method buns using half the amount of sugar. Carry out **sensory tests** on both recipes and compare your results.

- Suggest ways in which you could adapt a traditional recipe for cheese and bacon quiche to reduce the fat content. Make up your modified recipe and carry out a sensory analysis on the finished quiche.

- Give three ways in which the dietary fibre content of a traditional apple pie recipe could be increased. Make up your modified recipe and test it on your family.

Investigation

Group activity and class presentation

- Choose a selection of sweet and savoury recipes that would be suitable to serve at a birthday party for a six year old.

- Modify the recipes to reduce the fat, sugar and salt content, and increase the dietary fibre.

- Plan and make up the recipes as a group activity.

- Serve the party food, and carry out a sensory analysis of the finished products.

- Using a nutritional analysis program, compare the fat, sugar, salt and dietary fibre content of the original recipes with the modified ones.

Summary

Recipe balance is the combination of ingredients that gives a successful end product.

By modifying ingredients, the texture, taste and appearance of the product is changed.

Recipes can be made healthier by reducing the fat, sugar and salt content and increasing dietary fibre.

Convenience foods

What are convenience foods?

The term 'convenience foods' refers to foods which have been prepared or processed in some way. We mostly use convenience foods to save time, effort and in some cases money. Convenience foods can range from simple salad leaves, which have been washed and sealed in an airtight bag ready to serve, to a wide variety of ready made meals which just need reheating. There is a whole range of convenience foods available, which can be fresh, chilled, frozen, dried or canned.

A   *Types of convenience foods available*

Partly processed	Examples
The food manufacturer has carried out some of the preparation for you.	Ready diced, peeled or shredded vegetables, including stir-fry vegetable mixtures and salads
These can include fresh and chilled foods.	Most dishes with sauces, including pasta
	Fish pies, garlic bread, ready grated cheese, **cook-chill** chicken
Fully processed	**Frozen foods**
The food manufacturer has processed the food so that it can be defrosted, reheated or cooked with other foods.	Vegetables, burgers, fish, fish fingers, ready-meals, ice cream, desserts
	Dried foods
	Mashed potato, instant soup, gravy granules, baby rice, milk powder
(See 5.4, Food preservation.)	(some products need to be reconstituted with water or milk)
	Tinned foods
	Soups, vegetables, fruits, pie fillings, rice pudding, custard, fish such as tuna and sardines
	Jars
	Cook-in sauces, jam, baby food, pickles
Ready to eat	**Sweet**
	Biscuits, puddings, pies, mousses, snack bars, yogurts
	Savoury
	Cold meats, quiches, pasties, sausage rolls, meat pies, pizzas
Take-aways	
Although not strictly convenience foods, many people use take-aways in place of meals made at home.	Pizza, fish and chips, curries, Chinese meals, kebabs, sandwiches

Why are people using more convenience foods?

- Useful for busy people who have not got time to shop every day.
- More people own freezers and so are able to store ready prepared foods.
- More people own microwave ovens and are able to reheat ready prepared foods quickly.
- Change in shopping habits, particularly of families who tend to do a large shop periodically or shop online.
- Advances in food technology have improved the quality of convenience foods. For example, frozen pizzas, children's ready meals and luxury cook-chill ranges.

- Changes in meal patterns, with many families not eating at the same time.
- Increase in single person households, where it may be more economical to microwave a ready-meal than cook a meal from fresh ingredients.
- Useful for older people who may find it difficult to cook for themselves.

Disadvantages of convenience foods

- May be more expensive for families than making meals from fresh ingredients.
- Portions may be small, making it necessary to buy extra.
- Some products can be high in fat, sugar, salt and additives, although it is now possible to buy 'healthy ranges'.
- Eating too many processed foods limits the intake of dietary fibre.
- Excess packaging on convenience foods contributes to environmental damage.

Sensible use of convenience foods

- Combine convenience foods with fresh fruit and vegetables: for example, ready made pizza with green salad.
- Read the ingredients list on the packaging to check the fat, saturated fat, salt, sugar and fibre content.
- Do not eat convenience foods every day, or your diet may be very high in salt, fat and sugar and low in dietary fibre.
- Use ready made sauces in jars and packets to save time: for example, cheese sauce in lasagne or bolognese sauce with spaghetti.
- Frozen vegetables and fish retain their nutritional value and cook quickly.

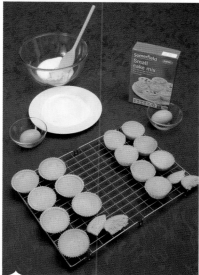

B   *Buns made from a packet mix compared with homemade*

AQA **Examiner's tip**

Remember to give a balanced answer on the advantages and disadvantages of convenience foods.

Investigation

- Visit your local supermarket (or look at a supermarket website) and make a list of all the different types of convenience food available.
- Test a range of ready made cake and pastry mixes, and compare them with the home made equivalents.

Practical activity

- Working in groups of four, make: 1 home made pizza; 1 pizza using a ready made base; 1 pizza using a packet mix base; and cook 1 frozen pizza.
- Carry out a sensory analysis and write a report on your findings.
- Compare the cost of each pizza.

Remember

Convenience foods can be part of a healthy diet if we eat lots of fresh foods as well.

Questions

1 What are convenience foods?

2 Name **three** different types of convenience food.

3 Give **three** advantages of convenience foods.

4 Give **three** disadvantages of convenience foods.

5 Describe ways in which convenience foods can form part of a healthy diet.

Summary

Convenience foods have been processed in some way.

Convenience foods save time and effort.

Convenience foods can be expensive for large families.

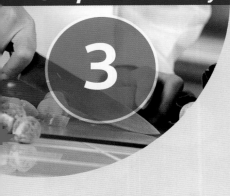

3

In this chapter you have learnt:

✔ the importance of storing food correctly

✔ how to avoid cross-contamination when storing raw and cooked foods

✔ how to organise time and resources in the kitchen, including the safe use of equipment

✔ why food is cooked and the different methods used for cooking food

✔ how recipes can be changed or adapted to make them healthier

✔ about the wide range of convenience foods available, and how you can combine convenience foods with fresh ingredients when preparing meals.

Revision quiz

1 Perishable foods should be stored in a:

a store cupboard

b refrigerator

c larder.

2 Non-perishable goods should be stored in a:

a store cupboard

b refrigerator

c freezer.

3 Which knife should be used for chopping onions?

a Bread knife

b Small vegetable knife

c Large cook's knife

4 Microwave ovens reduce cooking time when compared to conventional ovens by:

a up to 75 %

b up to 50 %

c up to 25 %.

5 When cooking food under the grill heat is transferred to the food by:

a conduction

b convection

c radiation.

6 When using a pressure cooker, heat is transferred to the food by:

a conduction

b convection

c conduction and convection.

7 The raising agent used in bread is:

a steam

b yeast

c baking powder.

8 The ingredient which shortens or tenderises recipes is:

a flour

b sugar

c fat.

9 Which of the following is classed as a convenience food?

a Garlic bread

b Milk

c Eggs

10 Which of the following statements is true?

a Convenience foods are unhealthy.

b Convenience foods have been processed in some way.

c Convenience foods are cheaper than using fresh ingredients.

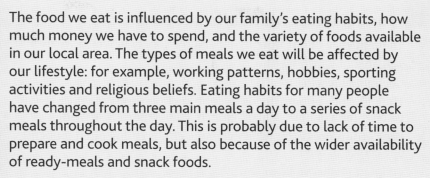

4

Factors affecting consumer choice

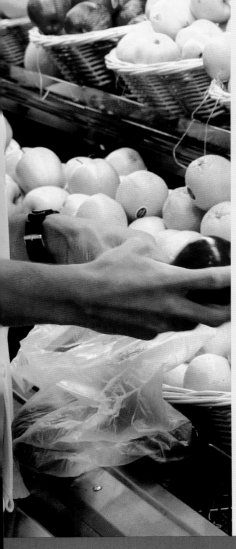

In this chapter:

4.1 Social factors affecting food choice

4.2 Economic factors affecting food choice

4.3–4.4 Factors affecting meal planning

4.5 Purchase of food

4.6 Choosing large kitchen equipment

4.7–4.8 Consumer issues and advertising

The food we eat is influenced by our family's eating habits, how much money we have to spend, and the variety of foods available in our local area. The types of meals we eat will be affected by our lifestyle: for example, working patterns, hobbies, sporting activities and religious beliefs. Eating habits for many people have changed from three main meals a day to a series of snack meals throughout the day. This is probably due to lack of time to prepare and cook meals, but also because of the wider availability of ready-meals and snack foods.

In this chapter you will learn about:

- the social factors which affect food choice, including cultural, religious, traditional and multicultural factors
- disposable income and its effect on the choices of food and cooking equipment
- the influence of changing lifestyles and family size on consumer choice
- the effects of the time available to buy and prepare food
- the factors which must be considered when planning meals for families including: special dietary needs; likes and dislikes; allergies and food intolerance
- the impact of technological advances in food production and cooking equipment on the types of food we eat
- the advantages and disadvantages of buying food at different types of retail outlet, including on the internet
- factors to consider when choosing and using electrical kitchen equipment
- the environmental impact caused by excessive packaging of food products and equipment
- the legislation involved in consumer protection
- the standards that must be met by manufacturers and retailers in the production and sale of food and related equipment
- advertising regulations, marketing and food promotion.

■ What you should already know:

✔ In Chapter 1 you learned about healthy eating guidelines which you should refer to when studying meal planning and the purchase of food.

✔ In Chapter 3 you learned about the organisational and practical skills that are required when preparing and cooking food.

Social factors affecting food choice

Social factors which affect food choice

- The influence of our upbringing and the family in which we live.
- The area in which we live.
- Changing lifestyles.
- The influence of our friends and the **social groups** to which we belong: for example, school, church, clubs, sporting activities.
- **Peer group pressure**: what everyone else is eating often influences our choice of food.
- Religious beliefs and festivals.

Objectives

Understand the influences of changing lifestyles and cultural norms on the choice of food and equipment.

Family background

Eating patterns are established from birth. Meal patterns, foods eaten, and the way in which they are eaten, are learned by children from their families. The types of food we like tend to be those which are liked by most of the family and are eaten often. As children grow older their eating habits change and they might develop food preferences which are different to those of their family.

Key terms

Social groups: friends or members of clubs, churches or organisations to which a person belongs.

Peer group pressure: conforming to what friends choose.

Where you live

If you live in a large town you have much greater access to a wide range of supermarkets and food outlets than if you live in the country. You will also have a greater choice of take-aways and fast-food restaurants. But in rural areas you may be able to buy more fresh foods from farmers' markets and farm shops.

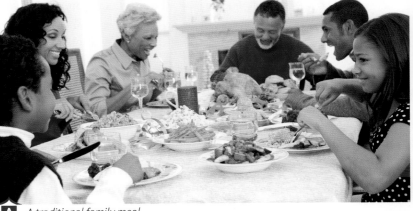

A _A traditional family meal_

Changing lifestyles

In families where both parents work there is less time for preparing meals and fewer families sit down together to eat an evening meal. People spend more time travelling to and from work, or work shifts, so it may not be convenient for them to eat together in the evening. Family members may also be involved in clubs and sporting activities after school or work, which can make it difficult for them all to eat at the same time.

Remember

The most important influence on food choices is family background.

Influence of friends and social groups

Children like to eat what their friends are eating in order to fit in. Teenagers, in particular, will eat pizza and drink fizzy drinks with their friends, even if they may not normally choose these foods. This is known as peer pressure. Adults will often choose to eat the same kind of food as their friends or they may recommend restaurants to other people in their social group.

AQA Examiner's tip

Ask your friends from different cultures about the foods they eat for special celebrations.

Religious beliefs and festivals

Our food choices may be affected by our religious beliefs which may not permit us to eat certain foods or at certain times. Religious festivals often involve eating traditional foods with our family and friends as part of the celebration.

B   *The influence of different religions on food choice*

Religion	Major festivals associated with food	Foods permitted/ forbidden
Buddhism	Wesak: when many Buddhists eat only vegetarian food and don't drink alcohol.	Many Buddhists do not eat meat.
Christianity	Christmas: when turkey, Christmas pudding, mince pies and Christmas cake are traditionally eaten. Easter: when hot cross buns, simnel cake and Easter eggs are traditionally eaten.	Does not forbid any foods, but some denominations eat fish on Fridays.
Hinduism	Diwali (Festival of Lights): often celebrated with a huge firework display and exchange of sweets.	Do not eat beef; many Hindus are vegetarian. Alcohol is forbidden.
Judaism	Passover: when a special meal is eaten, including unleavened bread (Matzah). Rosh Hashanah (Jewish New Year): when a special meal is eaten, including apples or bread dipped in honey. Yom Kippur (Day of Atonement): families eat before the sun sets, then fast for 24 hours. Hanukkah (Festival of Lights): when lots of delicious, and especially fried, foods are eaten.	Do not eat pork, shellfish or fish without scales. All food must be Kosher.
Islam	Ramadan: this is the ninth month of the Muslim calendar and lasts for a month. Fasting takes place during Ramadan from dawn to dusk. At the end of Ramadan there is a three day festival (Eid) when special foods are eaten.	Do not eat pork or fish without scales. Meat and poultry must be Halal. Alcohol is forbidden.
Sikhism	Guru Nanak's birthday: when Karah Parasaad, a sweet food made from flour, sugar and ghee is eaten.	Do not eat beef. Alcohol is forbidden.

C   *Jewish Passover food*

Investigation

- Working in groups, plan and make a celebration meal for a culture with which you are familiar.

- Research the multicultural influences on the modern British diet.

- Carry out a survey of school meals to identify the dishes that would be available to students with religious dietary restrictions.

Questions

1. What are the social factors that affect food choice?

2. How does where you live affect the variety of food available to you?

3. What effect have changing lifestyles had on our meal patterns?

4. How does peer group pressure affect the food choices of teenagers?

5. Give two examples of how food is related to religious festivals.

Summary

Food choices are mostly influenced by our families.

Changing lifestyles mean less time for preparing meals.

Children's food choices are influenced by their friends.

Food choices are influenced by religious beliefs.

4.2 Economic factors affecting food choice

Economic factors affecting food choice

These include disposable income, family size and spending patterns.

Disposable income

Disposable income is the amount of money people have to spend after they have paid taxes and other deductions. It is sometimes called 'take-home pay'. Budgeting for spending of take-home pay has to include bills such as rent or mortgage repayments, council tax and gas or electricity charges. The money left after these bills have been paid is used for food, clothes and luxuries such as holidays.

Although disposable income has risen since the 1980s the amount of money spent on food cooked at home has declined.

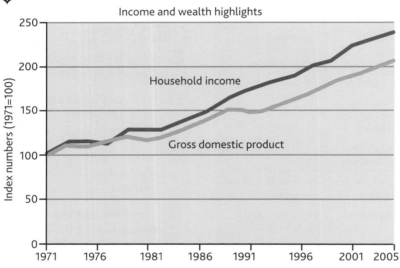

A *Changes in disposable income over time*

Real household disposable income and gross domestic product per head, UK

Source: National Statistics Online

Households with more disposable income tend to eat out more frequently; spend more money on premium ranges of ready prepared foods; and shop at more expensive supermarkets and specialist shops. Families with less disposable income tend to spend more on cheaper convenience foods and snack foods. Providing healthy meals for low income families requires careful budgeting and shopping around for cheaper prices.

Family size and spending patterns

Since the 1960s family size in Britain has been declining and there has been a sharp increase in single person households.

These changes are partly due to fewer children being born, but also to an **ageing population** and to more young, single people living alone.

Objectives

Understand the relationship between quality of diet and disposable income.

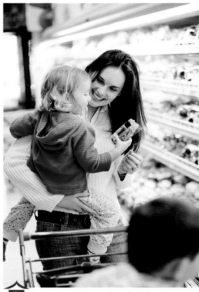

B *Shopping for the family's food*

Practical activity

- Plan, prepare and cook an economical dish that would be suitable for an evening meal for a low income family with two children.

- Work out the cost per portion of the dish.

Key terms

Disposable income: money left after tax and other deductions have been made.

Ageing population: a population where there are more elderly people than young people.

Expenditure on food varies with family size; with couples and single adult households spending more per person on food. As family size increases, less is spent per person on food. This could be because larger families include young children with smaller appetites, or because less food is wasted. It is possible to cook a meal such as shepherd's pie or lasagne for four people that does not cost much more than it would to cook the same meal for two. Larger families may also buy in bulk or shop around for cheaper prices or offers, such as three for the price of two, or buy one get one free.

C   *Changes in family size over time*

Households classified by size						
Households size	1961	1971	1981	1991	2003	2006
1 person	14	18	22	27	29	29
2 people	30	32	32	34	36	36
3 people	23	19	17	16	17	16
4 people	18	17	18	16	13	13
5 people	9	8	7	5	4	4
6 or more people	7	6	4	2	2	2
average household size	3.1	2.9	2.7	2.5	2.4	2.4

Source: Social Trends, Households classified by size

Food eaten away from home

Eating out has become a leisure activity and is no longer reserved for special occasions. There is a vast choice of places to eat out including: fast food chains; sandwich shops; pubs serving food all day; cafés at tourist attractions and leisure centres; and expensive restaurants and hotels for celebration dining. People with more disposable income eat out more frequently than those with less disposable income, but most people eat food outside the home on a regular basis.

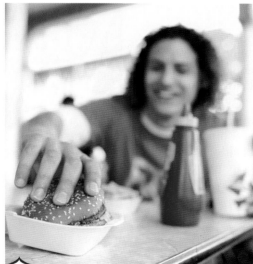

D   *Fast food restaurant*

Summary

Households with more disposable income spend more money on food than those with less disposable income.

Declining family size and an increase in single person households has led to a change in patterns of spending on food.

Questions

1 How does disposable income affect food choice?

2 Why is there an increase in people eating meals away from home?

3 Look at Table **C** and explain the trends in family size over the last 44 years.

4 How does family size affect food choice?

Planning family meals

The type of meals people eat at home depends on many factors.

- The budget available for food.
- The time and facilities available for preparing the food.
- The range of shopping facilities in the area, which affects the ingredients available.
- The skills of the cook.
- Family likes and dislikes.
- Special dietary needs of family members.
- Activities and hobbies of family members, which may result in meals being eaten at different times.
- The influence of celebrity chefs and television food programmes.
- The impact of food advertising.

Meal patterns

Snacking

Healthy eating habits are established in the home. The way we eat now has changed from the traditional meal pattern of three meals a day, where families would sit down together round a table. Today we are much more likely to eat small snacks throughout the day, which is known as **grazing**.

Most snacks consist of convenience foods, which are bought and consumed at break times, whilst travelling, in the office, or in public places. For people living alone, snacks may be more convenient and cheaper than cooking meals from fresh ingredients.

Snacks need not be unhealthy. It is possible to get individual salads in plastic containers, fresh fruit salads, yogurts with berries and muesli, and 'healthy' ranges of sandwiches. However, if you eat snacks frequently, check that they are low in fat, sugar and salt.

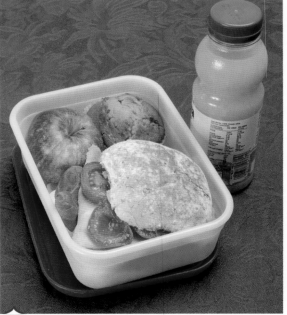

A *A healthy packed lunch*

Technological advances

Home freezers, microwave ovens, bread makers and food processors all save time in the preparation and cooking of foods.

New food products and the influence of advertising and the **media** increase our awareness of foods available.

Special dietary needs

Food related disorders

Some people are **allergic** to certain foods such as lactose in cow's milk; wheat; eggs; or certain additives such as monosodium glutamate or tartrazine.

The most serious allergy is to peanuts, and in some cases to nuts in general, which can cause a condition called **anaphylactic shock**. This is a very serious condition causing breathing difficulties, and the person can die if not given an injection of adrenalin immediately.

Coeliac disease is a condition where sufferers are sensitive to gluten in wheat and other cereal products. Wheat products are found in many foods, so it is important to check labels to make sure that they are gluten free.

Planning meals for toddlers and young children

Toddlers and young children can eat most foods that older children and adults eat, but they need much smaller quantities. They should be given a wide variety of fresh foods to provide their recommended intake of nutrients.

Meals for toddlers should be based on starchy foods such as potatoes, rice, pasta and bread; and include protein foods such as meat, fish, eggs and cheese; or vegetable proteins such as peas, beans, lentils and soya products. Vegetables and fruits should be included in their daily diet. Sugary snacks and drinks should be limited to prevent tooth decay. Yogurts, full fat milk and water can be given instead.

Planning meals for older children and teenagers

Older children and teenagers have increased energy, protein and calcium requirements, as they are going through a rapid growth period. Teenage girls require more iron once they start menstruation.

Healthy sources of energy for teenagers include pasta, rice, potatoes, bread (especially wholemeal) and wholegrain cereals. Milk, cheese, yogurt, bread and green vegetables will provide calcium for bone growth. Dark green vegetables (such as broccoli) fortified breakfast cereals, bread and meat will provide iron.

Planning meals for pregnant women

Eating healthily in pregnancy ensures that the unborn baby is adequately nourished and that the mother does not put on too much surplus weight, which may be difficult to lose once the baby has been born. Pregnant women should follow the 'healthy eating guidelines' (see 1.9) and normal family meals can be eaten during pregnancy.

However, while it is not necessary to 'eat for two', there is a need to increase energy foods, vitamin C and calcium during the last three months of pregnancy when the baby is growing rapidly. It is also particularly important to eat foods rich in dietary fibre, to prevent constipation.

With planned pregnancies, folic acid should be taken for three months before conception and for the first three months of pregnancy to prevent neural tube defects in the baby.

There are also some foods which should be avoided during pregnancy, which are listed opposite.

Questions

1. What is grazing?
2. Why are some snack foods unhealthy?
3. What are the points to consider when planning family meals?
4. Which foods should be avoided by pregnant women?

Planning meals for vegetarians

If one or more members of a family are vegetarian this has to be taken into account when planning and cooking meals. There are three main types of vegetarian:

Lacto-vegetarians

Lacto-vegetarians do not eat meat, poultry, fish or eggs; but will eat dairy products such as milk, yogurt, cheese and butter. Protein requirements can be met by mixing vegetable proteins such as soya (TVP), pulses and nuts, with milk, cheese and yogurt when planning meals.

Lacto-ovo-vegetarians

Lacto-ovo-vegetarians will eat dairy products and eggs, but not meat, poultry or fish. Protein requirements can be met as for lacto-vegetarians but with the addition of eggs.

Vegans

Vegans will not eat any foods from animals, including milk and eggs, or use any products, such as cosmetics, shoes or clothes, which use animal products. The main sources of proteins for vegans are soya products, pulses (peas, beans and lentils), nuts, seeds and cereals.

Planning meals for diabetics

Planning meals for diabetics should not be difficult as diabetics are advised to follow the same healthy eating guidelines as the rest of us.

People with insulin dependent (type 1) diabetes need to take daily injections of insulin to keep their blood sugar levels stable. People with non-insulin dependent (type 2) diabetes can control their blood sugar levels by following a healthy diet which is high in dietary fibre and low in sugar.

All diabetics need to eat regular meals and avoid missing meals or snacking on sugary snacks. Meals should be based on protein foods with plenty of vegetables and wholegrain starchy foods. Puddings and desserts can be sweetened with sweeteners rather than sugar; but fresh fruit, yogurts, or cheese and oatcakes are healthier choices for desserts.

Planning meals for people with coronary heart disease

Where a family member suffers from coronary heart disease (CHD), it is very important that the meals planned are low in **saturated fats**. These are the fats from animal sources (see 1.5), which contain more **cholesterol** than unsaturated fats, and can cause coronary arteries to become blocked.

Cholesterol is also made by the liver, but some foods which contain polyunsaturated fatty acids (PUFAs) reduce the production of cholesterol by the liver. Foods that contain PUFAs are oily fish such as salmon, mackerel, sardines, pilchards and herrings; and these foods should be included in meals for people suffering from CHD.

A diet rich in dietary fibre, from fruits, vegetables and wholegrain cereals, and low in saturated fat will help prevent the onset of heart disease.

Planning meals for weight loss

Where one or more family members are overweight, special attention has to be paid to the calorie content of the foods consumed. As we have seen in Chapter 1, if more food is eaten than is used up as energy, the result can be overweight and obesity. This can have very serious implications for health, as the risks of developing heart disease, type 2 diabetes, high blood pressure and joint problems increase when a person is overweight.

A recent government report found that levels of obesity have doubled during the last 14 years with 24 per cent of adults, 17 per cent of boys and 16 per cent of girls suffering from obesity. More than a third of the population is overweight, so these figures combined mean that over 50 per cent of the adult population is currently overweight or obese. (Source: the *guardian*, 17 December 2008, based on data from the NHS Health Survey for England, 2007.)

To maintain a healthy weight, we need to follow the 'healthy eating guidelines' (see 1.9) and increase physical activity to burn more calories. Meals should be planned using low fat ingredients, where possible, and extra fruit and vegetables should be included to add bulk to the diet. Snacks could include wholemeal bread, low fat yogurt, fruit, wholegrain cereals, or pasta with a low fat sauce. Sugary drinks should be replaced with water or diet drinks, to cut down on sugar consumption.

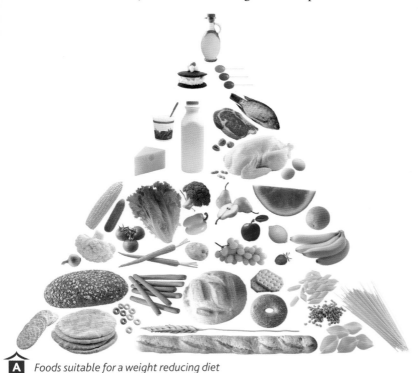

A *Foods suitable for a weight reducing diet*

Summary

The three main types of vegetarian are lacto-vegetarian, lacto-ovo-vegetarian, and vegan.

Type 2 diabetes can be controlled with a healthy diet.

To maintain a healthy weight we should eat a healthy diet and take more exercise.

Investigation 3

Heart disease

- What are the causes of heart disease and why is it increasing in Britain?

- Look on websites, e.g. the British Heart Foundation website, for comparisons with other countries.

- Interview a dietician about the dietary advice given to someone suffering from heart disease.

- Plan and make a main dish and a dessert for someone suffering from heart disease.

- Carry out sensory analysis of the dishes made.

- Carry out a nutritional analysis of the dishes and evaluate the saturated fat content.

∞ links

See Chapter 1 for more information about different dietary needs.

And take a look at the following websites:

The British Diabetic Association: www.diabetes.org.uk

The British Heart Foundation: www.bhf.org.uk

Investigation 4

Produce a range of leaflets and posters that give advice to young people about leading a healthy lifestyle to prevent obesity.

AQA Examiner's tip

Learn the different factors that influence meal planning.

4.5 Purchase of food

Retail outlets

Retail outlets are shops, large and small, where consumers can buy food and equipment that they need to provide meals for their families.

Objectives

Develop awareness of the different retail outlets available to consumers.

A *Advantages and disadvantages of different retail outlets*

Type of retail outlet	Advantages	Disadvantages
Hypermarkets	• Sell very wide range of products as well as food. • Competitive prices. • In-store facilities, such as: café, crèche, pharmacist, bakery, butchers and fresh fish counter. • Free parking. • Family friendly, with special trolleys and wide aisles. • Everything under one roof. • Cashback facility.	• Need a car to get there, as most are situated on the outskirts of large towns. • Cost of petrol has to be added to cost of shopping. • Takes a long time to go round very large hypermarkets. • May spend more than intended because of all the goods on offer.
Supermarkets	• Smaller than hypermarkets and can be local. • Quicker for doing a small shop. • Free parking. • Cashback facility. • Special offers.	• May not have as wide a range of goods as hypermarkets. • May be more expensive than hypermarkets. • Lack facilities such as café and pharmacy.
Specialist shops	• Wide choice of a particular type of food: e.g. meat at the butcher's, or fish at the fishmonger's. • Knowledgeable staff for advice or assistance. • Individual service. • Good quality of service. • Can buy as much or as little as you need.	• More expensive than supermarkets. • Fewer shops available. • May have to travel to get there. • Parking may be difficult.
Farmers' markets	• Fresh local produce. • Lower **food miles**, so environmentally friendly. • Free-range and **organic** produce available. • Food range changes with the seasons and availability.	• May have to travel to get there. • More expensive than supermarkets. • May only take place once a month. • Limited range of foods.
Corner shops	• Useful for the elderly, or people without cars who want to shop locally. • Stock most basic items, so useful for top-up shopping. • Open long hours. • Quicker than going to a large supermarket for a few items.	• More expensive than supermarkets. • May only sell a limited range of goods. • Fresh fruit and vegetables may be old or poor quality.
Internet shopping	• Saves time and effort for busy people. • Good for people without transport as goods are delivered to your door. • Able to select goods in the comfort of your home. • Can return goods if unsatisfactory.	• Need to have internet access and some IT skills. • Need to have a credit/debit card. • Cannot inspect goods before you buy. • May order more food than you require. • May be difficult to return unsuitable goods. • There may be a delivery charge.
Discount food stores	• Cheaper prices. • Value for money. • Free parking. • Useful for stocking up on basics.	• Smaller range of products to choose from. • Warehouse style shops in out of town areas, so need a car to get there.

Questions

1 Discuss the type of retail outlet that would be most suitable for a single person household.

2 Why is shopping for food on the internet becoming more popular for working parents with young children?

3 Compare the advantages and disadvantages of shopping for food at a discount food store with a supermarket.

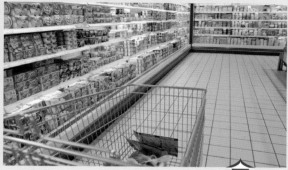

B *Supermarket*

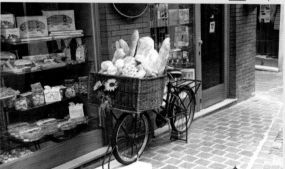

C *Specialist shop*

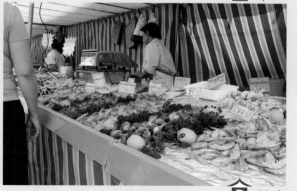

D *Market stall*

Key terms

Food miles: the distance food has travelled from harvesting, processing and packaging before it reaches the consumer.

Organic: foods that have been grown or reared without chemicals.

Investigation

Working in groups of four:

■ plan a weekly shopping list for basic items needed by four students sharing a house together.

■ using supermarket websites, compare prices for each item and work out which supermarket would give best value for the items needed.

Remember

Different methods of shopping suit different needs and resources.

AQA Examiner's tip

Try to give a balanced view of different methods of shopping with examples of people who would use each type.

Summary

Consumers can buy goods in many different types of shop.

Large supermarkets are generally cheaper than small shops, because they can buy products in vast amounts and have a large turnover.

Choosing kitchen equipment

Large pieces of kitchen equipment are expensive and are frequently used, so we need to carry out careful research before buying them. Useful information for consumers can be found in *Which?* reports and in magazines such as *Good Housekeeping*.

Cookers and microwave ovens

Types of cookers available

- Free-standing – as in range cookers.
- Built-in oven and separate hob.
- Combination cookers – which can have gas hobs, but electric or fan assisted ovens which use lower cooking temperatures. Other types of combination cookers may include a microwave oven in the design.

Factors to consider when buying a cooker

- The amount of cooking that is done in the household.
- The size of the family.
- The amount of money available – some cookers are very expensive, and you may not need all the additional features they offer.
- The type of fuel used – for example, gas, electricity or oil.
- Features required – such as self cleaning ovens or half grill features.
- Type of hob required – for example, gas burners, electric radiant rings, halogen rings, induction hobs or ceramic hobs.
- Safety factors – for example, cookers should have insulation to prevent the outside from getting very hot; electric cookers need a 30 amp electrical supply; gas cookers need to be fitted by a registered gas fitter.
- Free standing cookers can be moved if the owner moves house, but fitted hobs and ovens are usually left behind.

Factors to consider when buying a microwave oven

- Size of family and required uses – for example, defrosting, reheating, and cooking fresh ingredients.
- Space available in kitchen.
- Type required – for example, combination oven/microwave.
- Digital or manual controls.
- Design and style.
- Power output – can be from 500 watts to 1000 watts: the higher the power output the shorter the cooking time.

Refrigerators and freezers

Types of refrigerator available

- Larder fridge.
- Fridge with an small built-in ice box.
- Fridge/freezers.
- Free-standing or fitted into kitchen units.

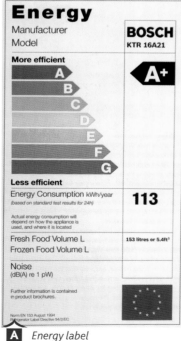

A *Energy label*

Factors to consider when buying a refrigerator

- Size of family – which will affect the **capacity** required.
- Additional features – such as ice makers, wine racks and automatic defrosting.
- Appearance – including colour and finish, such as stainless steel or aluminium.
- Amount of money available
- Running costs – check the **energy rating** on the label.

Factors to consider when buying a freezer

Similar to fridges but additional factors are:

- style of freezer – for example chest, or upright freezer with drawers.
- the type of food you are likely to freeze – home made or commercially frozen.
- the space available – chest freezers take up more floor space, so are better in a utility room or garage than in the kitchen.
- running costs – chest freezers are slightly cheaper to run than upright one.

Food processors, mixers and blenders

When buying food processors, mixers and blenders you should consider:

- how much preparation of fresh ingredients is done.
- required functions – for example, chopping, mixing, making dough, liquidising soup, or making smoothies.
- storage space available.
- additional attachments.
- ease of cleaning after use.
- cost and energy rating.

Safety factors when using electrical equipment

- Do not plug electrical equipment in with wet hands.
- Make sure flexes and wiring are not frayed or worn.
- Use oven gloves when removing hot pans and dishes from cookers and microwave ovens.
- Take care when washing sharp blades or slicing discs from food processors.
- Keep all equipment clean and free from grease and food particles in order to prevent food poisoning.
- Electrical kitchen equipment should carry one of the following safety labels: CE mark (European Union); British Electro-technical Approvals Board (BEAB); British Standards Institute (BSI) Kitemark.

Summary

Large pieces of kitchen equipment, such as fridges and cookers, should be chosen carefully, as they are used every day.

Information on electrical kitchen equipment can be found in *Which?* magazine.

Key terms

Capacity: storage size of fridges and freezers in litres.

Energy rating: how much energy an appliance uses: energy consumption, kWh/year.

Investigation

- Collect information on different types of cookers, fridges, freezers and microwave ovens.
- Evaluate each in terms of features, design, cost, energy rating and suitability for:
  - a a working family with two teenage children.
  - b a single person household.
  - c an elderly person who has frozen meals delivered.
- Present your results in a table.

Questions

1. What factors should be considered when buying a new cooker?

2. List the features that are available in modern refrigerators.

3. Discuss the advantages and disadvantages of a chest freezer.

4. What are the safety factors that must be considered when using electrical equipment?

▉ What is consumer protection?

Laws to make sure that the goods and services you buy are of a satisfactory quality and fit for purpose. When a consumer buys goods or services, they enter into a contract with the seller which is covered by **statutory regulations**. These are:

Sale and Supply of Goods Act 1994

This Act states that:

- goods must be of satisfactory quality, including safety aspects and materials used, and free from faults.
- goods must be fit for purpose: for example, a potato peeler must peel potatoes.
- goods must be as described on the packaging or in advertising.

Food Safety Act 1990

This Act covers all aspects of the food industry including the production, processing, storage, distribution and retail of food. Under the Food Safety Act, it is an offence to:

- sell food that could make people ill or that has been contaminated in some way.
- sell food that is unfit to eat.
- mislead consumers through exaggerated pictures or descriptions on labels, packaging or menus.
- sell food that is not of the quality described or make false claims about the nutritional value.

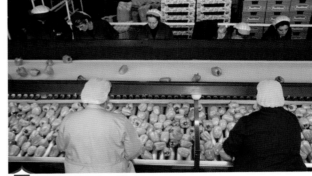

A   *Workers in a food factory*

Trades Descriptions Act 1968/72

This Act applies to second-hand goods as well as new products, and to items sold on the internet. It states that:

- goods must be described accurately by the seller; and the consumer must not be misled about the quality, price, manufacture, functions and safety aspects.

Weight and Measures Act 1985

This Act:

- protects consumers from goods being sold in incorrect weights and quantities: for example, pre-packaged meat must have the accurate weight and the price per kilogram on the label.
- states that packaged goods must show the exact weight of the contents on the packaging.
- ensures that where goods are sold loose and are weighed, for example fruit and vegetables, scales are checked for accuracy by Trading Standards Officers and traders can be prosecuted if scales are not accurate.

Remember

Although consumer legislation is in place to protect you when you buy goods and services, it is advisable to carry out consumer research before making expensive purchases.

AQA Examiner's tip

Know how the consumer is protected when buying goods and services.

Food Labelling Regulations 1995

Applies to processed and prepacked foods and states that labels should clearly show:

- name of the contents
- list of ingredients in descending order of weight
- address of the manufacturer
- use by date and best before date
- storage instructions
- weight of the food
- country of origin
- instructions for use.

Trading Standards departments of local authorities enforce these regulations.

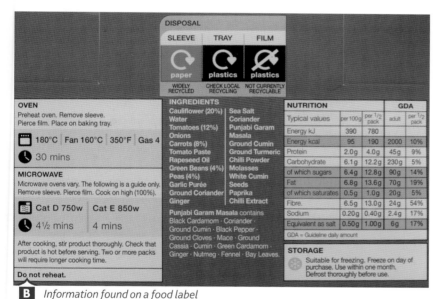

B *Information found on a food label*

Sources of advice for consumers

- The Trading Standards Department of your local authority can investigate false or misleading claims about, or concerns regarding the safety of, goods you have purchased.
- The Citizens' Advice Bureau (CAB) can give advice on individual complaints or about seeking **redress** in the Small Claims Court.
- The Environmental Health Department deals with complaints about unfit food or drink, such as nails in bread or beetles in flour, and dirty food shops and restaurants.
- The Office of Fair Trading is a government department which works to protect consumers from unscrupulous traders who try to deceive customers, or who provide unsatisfactory goods or services.
- Codes of Practice – most industries have voluntary 'codes of good practice' which responsible companies comply with.

Key terms

Statutory regulations: Acts of Parliament on which consumer law is based.

Redress: remedy, rectify or put right.

Questions

1 What is meant by consumer protection?

2 How does the Sale and Supply of Goods Act protect you when you buy a new microwave oven?

3 How does the Food Safety Act protect consumers when buying packaged food?

4 You have bought two kilograms of potatoes from a market stall but, when you get home and weigh them, you find you have only got one and a half kilograms. Who could you complain to, and which consumer legislation would cover your complaint?

Summary

Consumers are protected by legislation when buying goods and services.

The Food Safety Act covers all aspects of the food industry.

The Citizens' Advice Bureau is an independent organisation which can give information and advice on consumer issues.

Consumer issues and advertising 2

■ Complaining about faulty goods or services

Statutory rights state that you are entitled to a replacement or refund if:

- the product you bought was faulty or unsafe.
- the product was not as described on the packaging.
- the goods were not fit for the purpose intended.
- the product was not of a satisfactory standard.

You are not legally entitled to a replacement or refund if:

- you have changed your mind about the product.
- you have not followed the care instructions.
- you have damaged the product yourself.
- you have seen the product cheaper in another shop.

How to seek redress

- Take the product back to the shop where it was bought, with the receipt or other proof of purchase.
- Explain the problem, and if you don't get a satisfactory answer ask to speak to the manager (some large stores and supermarkets have customer service desks).
- If you fail to get a satisfactory outcome by speaking to the manager, write a letter of complaint to head office. You can find the address on the retailer's website.
- As a last resort you may decide to take your complaint to a Small Claims Court.

■ Advertising

Everywhere we go, we see advertising for different products and services: at the cinema; on buses and trains; on billboards; in shop windows; in newspapers, magazines and comics; on the television and radio; and on the internet.

Vast sums of money are spent on advertising, especially by manufacturers of convenience foods, crisps and snacks. Advertising is often aimed at children, as they can persuade parents to buy the products: this is known in the advertising industry as '**pester power**'.

How successful is advertising?

Very successful! Advertising can lead to massive increases in sales, particularly when products have celebrity endorsement.

New products have to be promoted to make the consumer aware of them, and this can be done in many ways: free samples; leaflets through the door; special offers; or **product placement** in supermarkets, sweets at the checkout, for example.

Advertising can be very subtle and incorporated into everyday life: for example, carrier bags that have the name and logo of the store; baseball caps from fast food chains; and pencil cases with drinks' logos on them.

Objectives

Develop understanding of methods of seeking redress.

Understand advertising strategies and regulations.

AQA **Examiner's tip**

Make sure you know the correct way to complain about faulty products or services.

Investigation 1 🔍

- Write a letter of complaint to a large retailer about a new cooker you have bought that has a faulty oven door.

- Describe the problem and say what you want done about it.

- What would be your next course of action if you failed to get a satisfactory response from the retailer?

Key terms

Pester power: children pestering adults to buy products.

Product placement: putting products in prominent places, such as at the end of aisles or at the checkout.

How is the consumer protected against misleading advertising?

Advertising Standards Agency (ASA)

This is an independent body which monitors and regulates the advertising industry through voluntary codes of practice. It covers advertising on posters; in magazines, newspapers and leaflets; on radio and television; and in cinemas.

It insists that advertising must be:

- legal
- decent
- honest and truthful.

Any individual can make a complaint to the ASA about advertisements that they think are indecent, dishonest, offensive or illegal. If the ASA upholds the complaint, they can refer the case to the Office of Fair Trading.

For example, in 2007, new rules on the advertising of foods aimed at children were introduced in response to concerns about increasing levels of childhood obesity. These rules state that advertisements for food products classified as high in fat, sugar and salt must not be shown during television programmes aimed at children under 16 years of age.

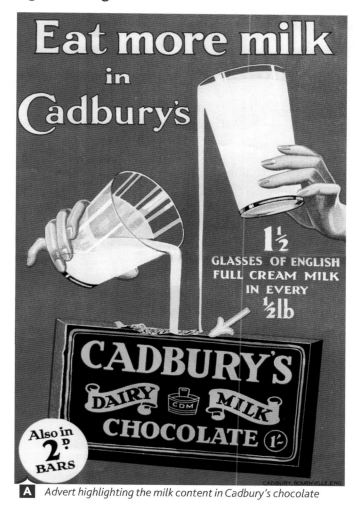

A   Advert highlighting the milk content in Cadbury's chocolate

Summary

You are legally entitled to a replacement or a refund if the product you bought was faulty or unsafe.

You are not legally entitled to a refund or replacement if you have changed your mind about a product.

Investigation 2

Collect different advertisements for convenience foods from magazines.

Make a table and record your comments on:
- who the product is aimed at
- what the manufacturer's claims are (for example, low in fat)
- whether or not you would buy it.

Questions

1 How is the consumer protected from misleading advertising for goods and services?

2 What is 'pester power' and how do manufacturers use it to sell more sweets and snack foods?

3 Describe how a new food product aimed at children might be marketed.

4 How would you make a complaint about misleading advertising?

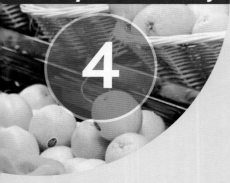

4

In this chapter you have learnt:

✔ how the food choices we make are influenced by social and economic factors

✔ that when planning meals for families, you must consider time, money, changing lifestyles and individual dietary needs

✔ that new technologies such as ready prepared meals, freezers and microwave ovens can influence meal planning

✔ that there is a wide range of different retail outlets available for the purchase of food and kitchen equipment

✔ how to carry out a consumer survey of large pieces of electrical equipment

✔ about the role of consumer legislation in protecting us when we buy goods and services.

Revision quiz

1 The most important factor that affects our choice of food is:
a where we live
b family background
c peer pressure.

2 Which of the following statements is true?
a Family size is increasing
b Family size is decreasing
c Family size has stayed the same for the last 50 years

3 Eating breakfast every day helps to:
a improve levels of concentration in children
b prevent coronary heart disease
c save money on snacks.

4 Which of the following foods should be avoided by pregnant women?
a Roast chicken
b Roast beef
c Fried liver

5 Which type of vegetarian will eat eggs?
a Lacto-ovo-vegetarian
b Lacto-vegetarian
c Vegan

6 When planning meals for coronary heart disease sufferers, which of the following fats should be reduced?
a Saturated fats
b Unsaturated fats
c Polyunsaturated fats

7 Shopping for food on the internet would be most be useful for:
a a single person household
b a household with teenage children
c a household where parents work full-time.

8 The most important factor to consider when buying a new cooker is:
a size
b colour
c the amount of cooking that is done in the household.

9 Consumers are protected from electrical goods which are faulty when purchased by:
a the Weights and Measures Act
b the Food Safety Act
c the Sale and Supply of Goods Act.

10 To make a complaint about a faulty product you should:
a phone the Trading Standards department of your local authority
b take it back to the shop where you bought it
c contact the Citizens' Advice Bureau.

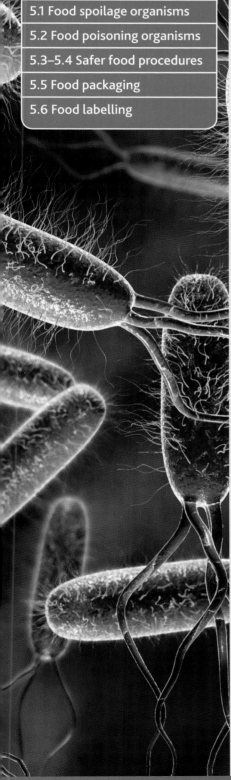

5 Food hygiene and safety

5.1 Food spoilage organisms

5.2 Food poisoning organisms

5.3–5.4 Safer food procedures

5.5 Food packaging

5.6 Food labelling

To make sure that the food we prepare and cook in the home is safe to eat, it is necessary to understand the sources of food poisoning and how contamination of food can be avoided by safe food handling practices.

In this chapter you will learn about:

- conditions that cause food poisoning
- the signs of food spoilage, including: enzymic action, mould growth, yeast production and bacterial contamination
- correct food storage to prevent contamination
- different types of food poisoning bacteria, including: *Salmonella, Listeria, Campylobacter, E coli, Clostridium perfringens* and *Bacillus cereus*
- high risk foods which are susceptible to food poisoning bacteria
- key methods for controlling food poisoning bacteria, including temperature control
- personal hygiene when handling, preparing, cooking, serving and reheating foods
- cross-contamination of raw and cooked food
- different methods of food preservation, including: freezing, cook-chill, dehydration, accelerated freeze drying (AFD), modified atmosphere packaging (MAP) and irradiation
- the different types and functions of food packaging, including: plastics, paperboard, foil and other metals
- the environmental implications of the use of excessive packaging materials
- the function of food labels and their advantages to consumers
- the statutory information that must appear on food labels.

■ What you should already know:

✔ In Chapter 2 you learned about the role of food additives which are used to preserve food and make it safe to eat.

✔ In Chapter 3 you learned about the importance of the correct storage of perishable and non-perishable foods, and in particular how you should store food in the fridge to prevent food poisoning.

✔ You also learned about the importance of hygienic use of equipment when preparing and cooking food, in order to prevent food poisoning.

Food spoilage

Food spoilage occurs when food is contaminated in some way, making it unsafe to eat. It is caused in different ways and can happen at any stage of the food production process. For example, physical contamination could take place from dirty machinery or careless food handlers. Food can also be contaminated by flies and vermin during transportation and storage.

Fresh food has a short shelf life and will start to decay soon after it reaches the shops. This is caused by enzymic action (see 2.1) and water loss. Further food spoilage is caused by the action of **micro-organisms**: the three main types are yeasts, moulds and bacteria.

Micro-organisms

Yeasts

These are tiny, single-cell fungi which can only be seen through a powerful microscope. Yeasts are found in the air and on the surface of some fruits.

Most types are harmless to humans and yeast is used to make bread rise. When it is mixed with sugar and kept warm it ferments producing carbon dioxide gas, and it is this gas that pushes up the structure of the bread causing it to rise. Yeast is also used to ferment grapes into wine, and hops into beer.

Yeasts are killed at temperatures above 100°C.

Moulds

Moulds are tiny plants which produce airborne spores. These can settle and grow on foods such as bread, jams, cheeses and soft fruits. Moulds can easily be seen as a blue fluffy growth on some foods. Moulds are used in the production of blue cheeses, to give them their characteristic flavour.

While most moulds are harmless, some produce toxins which are harmful to the body, which is why pregnant women should not eat blue cheeses.

Moulds grow in warm, damp conditions, so their growth can be prevented by storing foods in a refrigerator, especially in warm weather. Moulds can also be prevented by heating to high temperatures, as in jam making.

Bacteria

Bacteria are single-celled organisms which occur naturally in soil, air, water, and on humans and animals.

Bacteria need warmth, food, moisture, time and the correct pH in order to grow and multiply. Some bacteria also need oxygen to grow: these are known as **aerobic bacteria**. Others do not need a supply of oxygen, and can grow in the human intestines: these are known as **anaerobic bacteria**.

Bacteria multiply rapidly at temperatures below 63°C, but most are killed at temperatures of 72°C and above.

Objectives

Understand the conditions that cause food spoilage.

Did you know ??????

In order to grow and multiply micro-organisms need:

- warmth
- moisture
- food supply
- time
- air
- neutral pH.

If one or more of these conditions is removed then growth of micro-organisms is slowed.

AQA Examiner's tip

Be familiar with the causes of food spoilage and the conditions that micro-organisms need to grow and multiply.

Key terms

Micro-organisms: yeasts, moulds and bacteria.

Aerobic bacteria: bacteria which need oxygen to grow.

Anaerobic bacteria: bacteria which do not need oxygen to grow.

Remember

Bacteria multiply rapidly at temperatures between 5°C and 63°C.

Temperature control and the prevention of food spoilage

100°C – boiling point of water

72°C – safe reheating temperature

63°C – kills most bacteria but some
produce spores which
can survive this temperature

37°C – body temperature

} Danger zone

5°C – temperature in fridge:
bacteria dormant

0°C – freezing point of water:
some bacteria die, but others
remain dormant and become active
again once the food is thawed

A *Temperature control of bacteria*

Questions

1. List **four** conditions which bacteria need to multiply.

2. Give **three** uses of micro-organisms in food production.

3. Why are pregnant women advised not to eat blue cheeses?

4. What is the temperature 'danger zone' in which bacteria will multiply rapidly?

5. What happens to bacteria in food during freezing?

Outbreak of food poisoning after roast chicken lunch

A local restaurant serves carvery style Sunday lunches. One Sunday, the chef had forgotten to take the chickens out of the freezer the night before, so he tried to defrost them in the microwave. He then increased the cooking time of the chickens in the main oven by 20 minutes, before putting them on the hot serving counter for the 12.00 p.m. start of lunches. The last customer ate their chicken at 2.30pm. Later that day some of the people who ate the chicken started to feel ill, and by the next day 20 people were suffering from food poisoning.

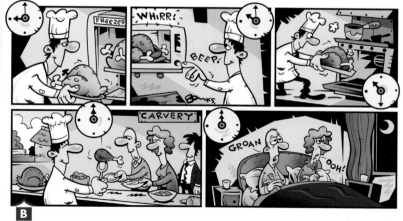

B

Case study

Questions

1. What were the possible causes of food poisoning in this case?

2. Name the bacteria that could have caused the food poisoning and the symptoms sufferers might have experienced.

3. How could this type of food poisoning be prevented in future?

Summary

The conditions needed for bacteria to grow are: warmth, moisture, food, the correct pH and time.

The temperature danger zone when bacteria will multiply is 5°C to 63°C.

A temperature of 72°C kills nearly all bacteria.

What is food poisoning?

Food poisoning is a common illness that is caused by eating foods that are contaminated with harmful bacteria. Contamination can occur at any stage during the production process. Food poisoning can occur if foods are not cooked at temperatures high enough to kill bacteria (above 72 °C); foods are handled by a person carrying bacteria; or foods are prepared in unhygienic conditions.

The symptoms of food poisoning usually include vomiting, diarrhoea, abdominal pains, headache, high temperature and fever. Many working days are lost each year because of people suffering from food poisoning.

The most common cause of food poisoning in the UK is contamination by **pathogenic bacteria**, including: *Salmonella, Campylobacter, E coli* and *Listeria*. Other bacteria which cause food poisoning are: *Clostridium perfringens* and *Bacillus cereus*, but these are much less common.

Objectives

Develop awareness of the different types of food poisoning bacteria.

Understand the key methods of control of food poisoning bacteria.

Key terms

Pathogenic bacteria: bacteria which are harmful to humans and can cause food poisoning.

Incubation period: the time between eating infected food and becoming ill.

AQA Examiner's tip

Make sure you understand methods of preventing and controlling food poisoning.

Case study

Read the following extract taken from a report in the *guardian* newspaper, 13 February 2008.

Families hit by *E coli* outbreak may bring case against butcher

Families of children who became ill during an outbreak of *E coli* that affected 150 people, mainly children, and claimed the life of one boy, could take legal action against the butcher blamed for the crisis, a public inquiry heard yesterday.

William Tudor was jailed over the outbreak, which affected 44 schools and left 31 children needing hospital treatment, but the Crown Prosecution Service decided not to bring a charge of manslaughter against him or his company.

On September 10 2005 the first symptoms of *E coli* 0157 were recorded in the South Wales valleys. Three children were admitted to Prince Charles hospital, Merthyr Tydfil, three days later.

An outbreak was declared on September 16, and it was not declared over until December 20. It was the largest outbreak of its kind in Wales, the second biggest in the UK, and the sixth largest worldwide.

It quickly became apparent that the young victims had all eaten school meals.

Cooked sliced meat supplied by the Bridgend butcher John Tudor & Son was soon identified as the common factor between the schools. When the premises were inspected, it was found that the the same set of scales and vacuum packing equipment was being used for both raw and cooked meat; and the vacuum packing machine was directly underneath an electric fly killer.

Symptoms suffered by the victims included vomiting and bloody diarrhoea. The poisoning can also lead to hallucinations and fits.

Questions

1 What were the causes of the food poisoning outbreak?

2 How many people were affected?

3 What were the symptoms experienced by the sufferers?

4 What precautions should the butcher have taken to prevent this outbreak?

A *Food poisoning: causes, symptoms and methods of control*

Food poisoning bacteria	Symptoms	Incubation period and duration	Causes	Methods of control
Salmonella	Vomiting, diarrhoea, nausea, headache, fever, abdominal pain	Incubation: 12–48 hours Duration: up to 7 days	• Infected poultry and eggs. • Cooked meats and pies. • Human and animal faeces.	• Thorough cooking above 72 °C to kill bacteria. • Food handlers should wear disposable gloves when serving cooked meats. • Wash and dry hands thoroughly after using toilet.
Campylobacter	Severe diarrhoea, abdominal pain, nausea, exhaustion	Incubation: 2–5 days Duration: 2–5 days	• Undercooked poultry and raw meat.	• Avoid cross-contamination from raw meat to cooked foods. • Cook poultry and meat to temperatures of 72 °C and above.
E coli (*Escherichia coli*)	Diarrhoea and passing blood, vomiting, dehydration *E coli* is very serious in babies, young children and the elderly Can lead to kidney disease and death	Incubation: 3–4 days Duration: can remain in intestines for long periods	• Raw meat and poultry. • Undercooked burgers and sausages. • Cross-contamination between raw and cooked foods. • Human and animal faeces.	• Defrost raw meat and chicken thoroughly before cooking. • Make sure they are cooked to 72 °C and above. • Wash and dry hands thoroughly after using toilet.
Listeria	Mild flu like symptoms Can invade bloodstream and cause brain disease Dangerous to pregnant women as it can cause stillbirth or miscarriage	Incubation: 5 days Duration: up to 5 weeks	Toxins found in: • water • manure and soil • soft cheeses and paté • unpasteurised milk • cook-chill products • prepared salads • cooked meats.	• Pregnant women should avoid soft cheeses, paté, and prepared salads. • Cooked foods should be stored below 5 °C. • Cook-chill products should be thoroughly reheated.
Bacillus cereus	Vomiting, diarrhoea, abdominal pain	Incubation: 2–18 hours Duration: 1–3 days	• Cooked rice and other grains.	• Avoid reheating – or keeping warm – cooked rice and other dishes containing grains.
Clostridium perfringens	Abdominal pains, diarrhoea	Incubation: 8–24 hours Duration: 12–24 hours	• Flies and bluebottles spread these bacteria. • Soil on vegetables. • Human and animal faeces. • Cooked meat dishes and pies which have been left out in a warm kitchen.	• Keep food covered to prevent contamination by flies. • Cool cooked foods rapidly and refrigerate as soon as possible. • Reheat foods thoroughly. • Avoid cross-contamination between raw and cooked foods. • Wash and dry hands thoroughly after using toilet.

Summary

Contamination of food can occur at any stage during the production process.

Symptoms of food poisoning include vomiting, diarrhoea and abdominal pains.

E coli poisoning is very serious and can cause death in babies, young children and elderly people.

■ Why are safer food procedures important?

Cases of food poisoning are increasing, and although there are many reasons for this, the main ones are:

- many more meals are being eaten outside the home, or bought as take-aways to be reheated at home.
- more ready prepared or convenience foods, which are reheated in the oven or microwave, are being eaten.
- foods are not being thoroughly cooked on barbecues.
- foods are not being kept at the correct temperature in the fridge or freezer.
- foods are being eaten after the best before or use by dates.
- cross-contamination between raw and cooked foods.
- the time taken from buying foods to placing in the fridge or freezer allows food poisoning bacteria to multiply.
- poor kitchen hygiene.
- poor hygiene of people who handle foods.

Objectives

Understand safer food procedures when selecting, storing and handling food.

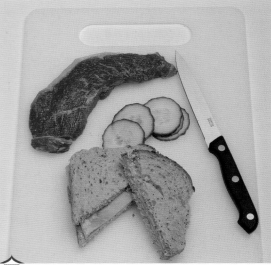

A *Cross-contamination of raw and cooked food*

Buying foods

- **High risk foods** such as cooked ham, chicken, shellfish, cooked egg dishes, cooked rice, and desserts containing cream, should be bought when needed and eaten before the use by date.
- Raw meat and poultry should be bought and used as needed or stored in a freezer.
- Frozen foods and high risk foods should be stored in a cool box when transporting home from the supermarket.
- Do not buy any packaged food that is damaged or leaking.

Storing foods

- Chilled foods should be stored in the fridge at temperatures from 0–5 °C.
- Cooked foods should be stored in the fridge above raw foods, to avoid cross-contamination (see 3.1).
- Foods stored in the fridge need inspecting frequently for decay and to check that they are within their use by dates.
- Fridges should be kept clean and a fridge thermometer used to check the temperature.
- Do not overload the fridge, as air needs to circulate to keep the food cool.

Remember

High risk foods, which are most susceptible to food poisoning, are chicken, shellfish, eggs, and desserts containing cream.

AQA *Examiner's tip*

Make sure you know how to store foods correctly in the fridge and freezer.

- Do not put warm food in the fridge as it raises the temperature.
- Frozen foods should be stored in freezers at temperatures below -18°C.
- When freezing fresh food in a domestic freezer, do not put too much in at once, as this will raise the freezer temperature and increase the time it takes the food to freeze.
- Do not refreeze food once it has been defrosted.
- If raw meat or fish becomes defrosted, for example after a power cut, it can be cooked and refrozen, but should be used up as soon as possible. Cooked foods should be thrown away and not refrozen.
- For foods stored in cupboards or a larder, it is important to check the best before dates and make sure that the oldest food is used first. This is known as **stock rotation** and prevents dry goods, such as flour, from becoming rancid or infested by beetles.

> ### Key terms
>
> **High risk foods**: foods which are easily contaminated with food poisoning bacteria.
>
> **Stock rotation**: checking best before dates on dry goods and using the oldest first.

Handling and preparing food

High standards of personal hygiene are very important when handling and preparing food in the home.

B *Hygiene rules for food handlers*

Hygiene rules for food handlers	Reasons
• Always wash your hands with hot soapy water and dry them thoroughly before handling food and after using the toilet.	• Bacteria on your hands can be transferred to food.
• Do not cough or sneeze over food, and wash your hand after blowing your nose. • Do not lick your fingers or use cooking utensils for tasting.	• Many bacteria live in the nose and throat and can be transferred to the food.
• Make sure cuts and sores are covered with waterproof dressings.	• Bacteria can live in cuts and sores and can be transferred to food.
• Wash your hands after handling raw meat and poultry.	• Bacteria in meat and poultry can be transferred to your hands and on to other foods.
• Wear a clean apron.	• To prevent contamination from bacteria on your clothes.

Questions

1. Why are cases of food poisoning increasing?

2. What precautions should you take when buying and storing high risk foods?

3. What should you do if food in your freezer thaws after a power cut?

4. Why is it important that food handlers should wash their hands after blowing their nose or visiting the toilet?

Investigation

Design a leaflet or poster with information on safe food procedures for ONE of the following:

- Buying food
- Storing food
- Handling food
- Preparing food

Summary

Foods should be bought from shops with high standards of food hygiene.

Foods should be stored correctly in the home to prevent bacteria multiplying.

Food handlers should have high standards of personal hygiene.

5.4 | Safer food procedures 2

Food preparation areas

- Work surfaces, sinks and cookers should be kept clean by washing with hot soapy water or an **antibacterial** cleaner.
- Fridges should be washed out frequently with hot soapy water and rinsed with clean water.
- Freezers should be defrosted as required and washed, as fridges.
- All cooking utensils should be kept clean and free from food deposits.
- Prepare raw and cooked foods on separate chopping boards, to avoid cross-contamination.
- Dishcloths and tea towels should be cleaned and **sterilised** frequently. Dishcloths can be sterilised by placing in the microwave for one minute.
- All food must be kept covered to avoid contamination from flies.

Serving and reheating food

- Food should be served as soon as possible after it has been cooked.
- If food is kept warm, it must be kept over 63 °C and for no longer than 20 minutes to avoid bacterial contamination.
- Food that is going to be reheated should be cooled rapidly and refrigerated as soon as possible.
- When food is reheated in a microwave, make sure that it is heated right through and that there are no cold spots. A food thermometer is useful for testing reheated food.

■ Food preservation

Why is food preservation necessary?

Food is preserved to prevent decay, and keep it safe to eat for longer periods than it would be in its natural state. Preservation can be short term, for example chilling and cooking food; or long term, for example drying and freezing.

Objectives

Understand safer food procedures when preparing, cooking and serving food.

Understand the scientific principles involved in food preservation.

Key terms

Antibacterial: prevents bacteria from spreading.

Sterilisation: a heating process which kills bacteria.

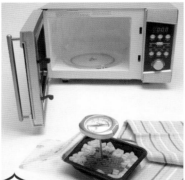

A *Checking the temperature of food reheated in a microwave*

Practical activity

- Carry out a comparison of home made, tinned and packet soups.
- Set up a taste panel to test the soups and record your results in a table.

Questions

1. Why is food preservation necessary?
2. Explain how the removal of water preserves food.
3. Give examples of foods which are suitable for canning.
4. What are the effects of freezing on the nutritional value of meat and vegetables?
5. What are the disadvantages of freezing as a method of food preservation?
6. Why are flavourings added to dried soups and snack meals?

Summary

Food preparation and storage areas should be kept clean and free from bacterial contamination.

Hot food should be kept at temperatures above 63 °C to keep it safe to eat.

Food preservation prevents decay.

B *Scientific principles of food preservation*

Method	Action	Suitable foods
Removal of water (drying)	Prevents enzymic activity and micro-organisms from causing decay.	Milk powder, coffee, vegetables, pulses, soups, instant snacks
Heating (canning, bottling, pasteurisation of milk)	Destroys micro-organisms and enzymic activity.	Fruit, vegetables, soups, beans, pasta in sauce, fish, meat, milk, cream
Reduction of temperature:		
Freezing	Micro-organisms and enzymes dormant during freezing.	Fish, meat, vegetables, ready-meals, pies, pizza
Chilling	Reproduction of micro-organisms slowed down during chilling.	Ready-meals, salads, desserts, pizza, sandwiches
Use of chemicals (such as salt, vinegar and sugar)	Destroys micro-organisms and inhibits enzymic activity.	Vinegar – pickled vegetables, chutneys, olives Salt – salted snacks Sugar – jam and marmalade
Removal of air (vacuum packing, modified atmosphere packaging [MAP])	Without air micro-organisms cannot multiply.	Bacon, cheese, sausages, cooked fish, crisps, paté, cooked meats
Irradiation	Radiation treatment kills micro-organisms (it does not make food radioactive).	Potatoes, shellfish, spices, pulses, fruits (in particular strawberries, bananas and mangoes)

C *Effects of different methods of preservation on nutrient value of food*

Method	Foods treated	Effect on nutritional value
Heat treatment: Sterilisation (heating to 132 °C) Pasteurisation (heating to 72 °C)	Milk, canned and bottled foods Milk, milk used for yogurts and cheese	• Destroys heat sensitive vitamins such as thiamin and vitamin C. • Lactose is partly caramelised which alters the flavour of sterilised milk.
Dehydration including accelerated freeze drying (AFD), where food is frozen first before the ice crystals are removed in a vacuum	Milk, instant potato, coffee, tea, fish, meat, vegetables, pulses, herbs, soups, instant snack meals	• Heat sensitive and water soluble vitamins lost (thiamin and vitamin C). • Freeze dried foods retain more vitamin C than traditional drying methods. • Loss of flavour and texture in dried foods are often compensated by the addition of flavouring ingredients. • Some dried foods have more concentrated flavours, e.g. dried onions and fruits.
Chilling – chilling temperature (domestic fridges) is normally 5 °C	Fresh meat, fish, cooked meat, eggs, green vegetables, salads	• Water soluble vitamins B and C lost as food dries out in fridge.
Freezing – freezing temperature is normally: –18 °C in domestic freezers –34 °C for foods frozen commercially	Vegetables, fish, meat, ready-meals, ice cream, fruits such as berries and apple slices	• Some loss of vitamins B and C when vegetables are blanched prior to freezing. • Loss of protein and B group vitamins when fresh meat thaws prior to cooking.
Use of chemicals (pickling, salting and jam making)	Vegetables, chutneys, fish, meat, fruits (for jam)	• Where heat treatment is involved in the processing, thiamin and vitamin C are lost. • Vitamin C is also lost from fruits when making jam.

5.5 Food packaging

◼ Why do food manufacturers use food packaging?

- To **protect** food from damage during transportation and storage.
- To keep food in good condition and **preserve** freshness: for example, tomatoes and strawberries in plastic boxes.
- To **prevent** contamination from dust, flies and bacteria.
- To **inform** consumers about the product.
- To **enhance** the appearance of products.

Different types of packaging

Plastics

Plastics are very versatile packaging materials and can be used for a wide range of foods including: milk; yogurts; drinks bottles; fruit and vegetable boxes; ready-meals, including microwavable meals.

Advantages – lightweight and waterproof; can be moulded or shaped; can be clear or coloured; can be printed with information; can be used for vacuum packing.

Disadvantages – not as strong as glass or metal; made from hydrocarbons, which are in limited supply and expensive; although some are recyclable, others are not, and have to be disposed of in landfill sites.

Paperboard

Paperboard is increasingly used for cook-chill ready-meals, salads and sandwiches. Fruit juices are sealed in waxed paperboard or polyethylene cartons in a process called aseptic packaging.

Advantages – strong; lightweight; made from renewable sources; can be recycled.

Disadvantages – not as strong as plastic and will crush easily; not moisture proof, so food will dry out during storage.

Metals

Aluminium containers are used widely for ready-meals and canned drinks. Canned food is one of the oldest methods of food preservation and is used for a wide variety of foods including fruits, vegetables, fish, meat, soups, custard and rice pudding.

Advantages – strong and rigid, giving good protection to the food; canned food can be stored for a long time; metals used are recyclable.

Disadvantages – cannot put metal containers in the microwave; production process uses a lot of energy.

Glass

Glass is widely used for packaging jams, pickles, chutney, sauces, baby food and milk.

Advantages – rigid and moisture proof so gives good protection to the food; can be recycled.

Disadvantages – brittle, easily broken and heavy.

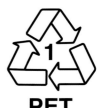

A *Plastics that can be recycled have this symbol on the packaging*

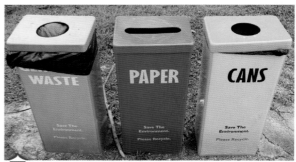

B *Recycling bins*

New developments in packaging

Manufacturers are constantly developing new types of packaging to make food more appealing to the consumer and safer to eat. These include:

tamper-proof seals on, for example, baby food, jam jars and squash bottles. These prevent deliberate contamination of food and reassure consumers about its safety.

ring-pull cans for soups, drinks, vegetables and fruit. These are easier to open for elderly or disabled people.

vacuum packaging which is used for coffee, bacon and cheese. This method removes the air so the product will keep for longer.

modified atmosphere packaging (MAP) which is used for ready-meals, meat, fish and salad leaves. Oxygen is removed from the packaging and replaced with an inert gas such as carbon dioxide or nitrogen. This slows down food spoilage and the development of micro-organisms.

Questions

1. List **four** reasons why food manufacturers use food packaging.

2. What are the advantages and disadvantages of using plastics for packaging?

3. What is MAP?

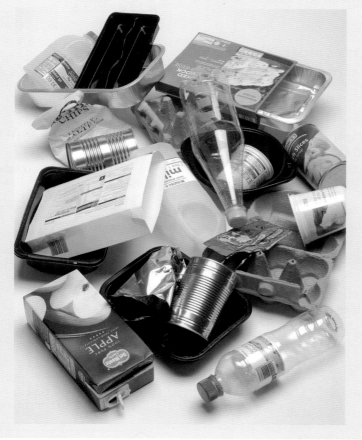

C *Packaging materials*

Key terms

Tamper-proof seals: plastic collars on lids and shrink-wrapped jars to ensure that foods have not been contaminated.

Vacuum packaging: plastic packaging where all the air has been removed.

AQA Examiner's tip

Be familiar with a range of food packaging materials, and be able to give examples of how they are used.

Investigation

- Make a collection of different packaging materials and compare: the uses; the food they contained; how necessary the packaging was to the freshness and safety of the food.

- Find out what major food manufacturers are doing about excessive packaging, and make suggestions as to how waste from packaging could be reduced.

∞ links

For further information and advice about recycling go to:

www.recyclenow.com

Summary

Packaging is used to: protect and preserve food; prevent contamination; inform consumers; enhance appearance.

Plastics are made from hydrocarbons, which are becoming scarce.

Production processes for metal containers use a lot of energy.

■ What are the functions of food labels?

Manufacturers use food labelling on processed food to pass on information to the consumer. The Food Labelling Regulations (see 4.7) control what information manufacturers have to put on food labels.

Advantages to consumers

Labels enable consumers to make informed decisions about the food they buy. The label will give information on what is in the product and the amount of each ingredient; the date mark will tell the consumer how long the product is safe to eat; and the storage and cooking instructions give further information to prevent food poisoning.

Labels must show:

- the full name of the product, including any treatment it has had (for example UHT milk or smoked salmon).
- the ingredients list, including additives, in descending order of weight.
- the weight of the product with the letter **e** which means that the average weight must be accurate.
- the shelf life, including the best before date on processed food and the use by date on fresh foods.
- storage instructions.
- the name and address of the manufacturer, packer or retailer.
- the place of origin of the product, for example coffee from Kenya.
- instructions for use.

Optional information includes:

- nutritional information, including comparisons with **GDAs** for calories, sugars, fat, saturated fat, and salt per serving.
- **allergy** information.
- suitability for vegetarians.
- special claims, such as enriched with calcium.
- bar code for stock control.
- recycling information.

Traffic light labelling

- A growing number of supermarkets and food manufacturers are using traffic light colours on the labels to help consumers make healthy food choices.

Investigation 🔍

Find out:
- ■ what the traffic light labelling colours mean
- ■ where you would find them
- ■ how they can help you make healthy food choices.

Objectives

Understand the functions of food labelling.

Remember

The function of food labels is to inform the consumer about the product and how to store and use it.

AQA Examiner's tip

Make sure you know the statutory information that must appear on a food label.

Key terms

GDA: guideline daily amount of nutrients.

Allergy: adverse reaction to certain ingredients in foods.

∞ links

For more information about traffic light labelling go to:

www.eatwell.gov.uk/foodlabels/trafficlights

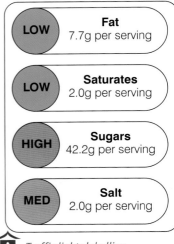

LOW	**Fat** 7.7g per serving
LOW	**Saturates** 2.0g per serving
HIGH	**Sugars** 42.2g per serving
MED	**Salt** 2.0g per serving

A Traffic lights labelling

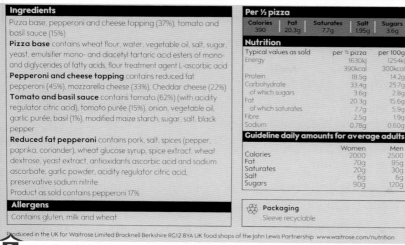

Ingredients
Pizza base, pepperoni and cheese topping (37%), tomato and basil sauce (15%)
Pizza base contains wheat flour, water, vegetable oil, salt, sugar, yeast, emulsifier mono- and diacetyl tartaric acid esters of mono- and diglycerides of fatty acids, flour treatment agent L-ascorbic acid
Pepperoni and cheese topping contains reduced fat pepperoni (45%), mozzarella cheese (33%), Cheddar cheese (22%)
Tomato and basil sauce contains tomato (62%) (with acidity regulator citric acid), tomato purée (15%), onion, vegetable oil, garlic purée, basil (1%), modified maize starch, sugar, salt, black pepper
Reduced fat pepperoni contains pork, salt, spices (pepper, paprika, coriander), wheat glucose syrup, spice extract, wheat dextrose, yeast extract, antioxidants ascorbic acid and sodium ascorbate, garlic powder, acidity regulator citric acid, preservative sodium nitrite
Product as sold contains pepperoni 17%
Allergens
Contains gluten, milk and wheat

Per ½ pizza

Calories	Fat	Saturates	Salt	Sugars
390	20.3g	7.7g	1.95g	3.6g

Nutrition

Typical values as sold	per ½ pizza	per 100g
Energy	1630kJ	1254kJ
	390kcal	300kcal
Protein	18.5g	14.2g
Carbohydrate	33.4g	25.7g
of which sugars	3.6g	2.8g
Fat	20.3g	15.6g
of which saturates	7.7g	5.9g
Fibre	2.5g	1.9g
Sodium	0.78g	0.60g

Guideline daily amounts for average adults

	Women	Men
Calories	2000	2500
Fat	70g	95g
Saturates	20g	30g
Salt	6g	6g
Sugars	90g	120g

Packaging
Sleeve recyclable

Produced in the UK for Waitrose Limited Bracknell Berkshire RG12 8YA UK food shops of the John Lewis Partnership www.waitrose.com/nutrition

B Nutritional information shown on a frozen pizza box

Labels must not make misleading claims

- The picture on the packet must represent the food inside. So if, for example, a ready-meal shows two chicken breasts in sauce with vegetables on the packet, then it must contain two chicken breasts, sauce and vegetables.

- Fruit yogurts and desserts must contain the fruit described on the label. So if, for example, the label says 'black cherry yogurt' then it must contain black cherries. If, however, the yogurt is flavoured with additives and does not contain any fruit, then it must be called 'black cherry flavoured yogurt' on the label.

- Products must not claim to be 'reduced' fat if they do not contain less fat than the standard version or 'low fat' if they contain more than 3 g of fat per 100 g.

- Products must not claim to contain extra nutrients, for example high fibre bread or high calcium milk, if they do not contain more than the normal version.

- Products must not claim to be suitable for vegetarians if they contain any animal flesh (meat, fish, fowl or shellfish) or any ingredient resulting from slaughter.

Kellogg's® COCO POPS®

Allergy Information
Contains Barley.

Nutrition Information

	Typical value per 100 g	Per 30 g serving with 125 ml of semi-skimmed milk
ENERGY	1641 kJ 387 kcal	743 kJ 175 kcal
PROTEIN	5 g	6 g
CARBOHYDRATE	85 g	32 g
of which sugars	36 g	17 g
starch	49 g	15 g
FAT	3 g	3 g
of which saturates	1.5 g	2 g
FIBRE	2 g	0.6 g
SODIUM	0.45 g	0.2 g
SALT	1.15 g	0.5 g

VITAMINS:		(% RDA)		(% RDA)
THIAMIN (B_1)	1.2 mg	(83)	0.4 mg	(29)
RIBOFLAVIN (B_2)	1.3 mg	(83)	0.7 mg	(44)
NIACIN	14.9 mg	(83)	4.7 mg	(26)
VITAMIN B_6	1.7 mg	(83)	0.6 mg	(29)
FOLIC ACID	166 µg	(83)	58 µg	(29)
VITAMIN B_{12}	0.83 µg	(83)	0.77 µg	(77)
MINERALS:				
CALCIUM	456 mg	(57)	288 mg	(36)
IRON	8 mg	(57)	2.4 mg	(17)

A 30 g serving of Kellogg's Coco Pops provides at least 25 % of the recommended daily allowance (RDA) of the vitamins thiamin, niacin, vitamin B_6, riboflavin (B_2), vitamin B_{12}, and folic acid; and 17 % RDA of the minerals iron and calcium.

Kellogg Marketing and Sales Company (UK) Limited, Manchester M16 0PU.

© 2007 Kellogg Company
® Kellogg Company

PIN: K115775002

C Legal and optional information found on packaging

Questions

Look at the nutrition information on the pizza label **B** and answer the following questions.

1 What is the percentage GDA of fat for a man provided by half the pizza?

2 Is this product high or low in fat?

3 What other foods could be eaten with the pizza to increase the nutritional value?

Summary

Labels provide information to enable consumers to make informed choices when buying food.

Labels give information on safe storage and cooking to prevent food poisoning.

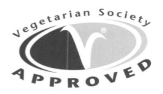

Vegetarian Society APPROVED
www.vegsoc.org

D This symbol shows the food is suitable for vegetarians

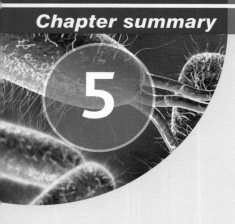

Chapter summary

5

In this chapter you have learnt:

✔ about the conditions that cause food spoilage and how it can be prevented

✔ what food poisoning is, and how it is caused

✔ that it is important to follow safe food procedures when handling and cooking food

✔ why foods are preserved and the different methods of food preservation

✔ the properties of different types of food packaging materials and the functions of each type

✔ about the information available to consumers on food labels.

Revision quiz

1 How might food be contaminated if it is left uncovered in the kitchen?

a By sunlight

b By flies

c By dirty machinery

2 The critical points between which bacteria multiply are:

a 5–63°C

b 0–72°C

c 5–100°C.

3 Food poisoning is caused by:

a enzymes

b pathogenic bacteria

c yeasts.

4 Which of the following foods is classed as high risk for causing food poisoning?

a Cooked chicken

b Fried fish

c Pizza

5 The temperature of a fridge should be:

a 0–10°C

b 0–15°C

c 1–8°C.

6 The process of heating milk to remove harmful bacteria is known as:

a caramelisation

b pasteurisation

c homogenisation.

7 The process of removing water to preserve foods is known as:

a sterilisation

b vacuum packing

c dehydration.

8 Most plastic packaging materials are made from:

a polyester

b hydrocarbons

c cellulose.

9 Which one of the following items of information has to be on a food label by law?

a V symbol for vegetarians

b Nutritional information

c Weight of the product

10 Labels on perishable foods should include:

a use by date

b best before date

c best before end date.

6   Controlled Assessment

6.1   How Controlled Assessment works

Objectives

Understand the Controlled Assessment part of your course.

Understand how you will be assessed.

AQA Examiner's tip

Controlled Assessment makes up 60 % of the total mark so it's very important that you produce your best possible work.

What is Controlled Assessment?

Controlled Assessment used to be called coursework. It is now made up of two tasks:

1   An **Individual Investigation** which is worth 45 % of the total mark and on which you should spend approximately 18 hours.

2   A **Research Task** which is worth 15 % of the total mark and on which you should spend approximately 6–8 hours.

Both tasks must be completed on A4 paper.

When will I do the Controlled Assessment?

A range of tasks will be provided, by AQA, for both the Investigation and the Research Task at the start of the academic year. It is advised that you will complete the Research Task towards the end of Year 10 and the Individual Investigation in Year 11. In both tasks you will need to show your knowledge and understanding of the subject content of the specification. You will also need to show your skills and knowledge in: planning and carrying out investigations using appropriate research methods; analysing and evaluating information; making reasoned judgements; and presenting conclusions.

How is it assessed?

The three assessment objectives are shown in Table **A**.

A Assessment objectives for the Controlled Assessment

Assessment objective	Areas covered
AO1 (10 % of marks) Recall, select and communicate their knowledge and understanding of a range of contexts.	• Identify issues and questions. • Assemble relevant information.
AO2 (40 % of marks) Apply skills, knowledge and understanding in a variety of contexts and in planning and carrying out investigations and ideas.	• Task analysis. • Analyse information. • Identify a clear course of action. • Plan a practical solution based on the evidence gathered. • Carry out the practical work, demonstrating a wide range of appropriate skills/processes.
AO3 (10 % of marks) Analyse and evaluate information, sources and evidence; make reasoned judgements and present conclusions.	• Evaluate research, practical work, sensory and nutritional analysis. • Interpret the evidence with reference to the issues identified in the task analysis. • Produce a report on the conclusions drawn from the investigation.

6.2 Individual Investigation

What will I have to do for the Individual Investigation?

- Choose a topic from the list provided by AQA.
- Carry out a task analysis of the topic, to identify areas that you might research. (See example **A** for how this could be done.)
- Research background information on the areas identified.
- Use a variety of **primary** and **secondary** research methods.
- Analyse the information gathered and identify the main issues (problems) that you will try to solve.
- Produce a clear statement of aims (what you intend to do) with justifications (why you are doing it).
- Plan practical solutions based on your research analysis. Justify your choice of dishes with reasons linked to your research.
- Aim to spend at least 6 hours on practical work. Try to show as wide a range of food preparation and cooking skills as possible, and pay attention to food safety and hygiene.
- Produce time plans and recipes to show how your practical work will be organised.
- Make sure your finished dishes look colourful and attractive.
- Carry out sensory analysis (see 2.3 and 6.3) on some of the dishes made, so that you can discuss the colour, taste and texture of the food in your evaluation.
- Carry out nutritional analysis (see 6.3) of the dishes made and work out costs where appropriate.
- Present your results in tables and graphs with comments on the findings.
- Photograph your finished dishes to put in your folder.

Objectives

Understand how to approach the Individual Investigation part of your Controlled Assessment.

Understand how to evaluate your Investigation.

Key terms

Primary research: information that you find out for yourself.

Secondary research: information that someone else has produced: for example, books, leaflets, magazines, newspaper articles and websites.

Investigation

Example of an Individual Investigation

Many young people living away from home, e.g. students, rely on take-away food and ready-meals. Investigate and make a range of nutritious dishes that would:

- be economical
- be easy to make
- satisfy their dietary requirements.

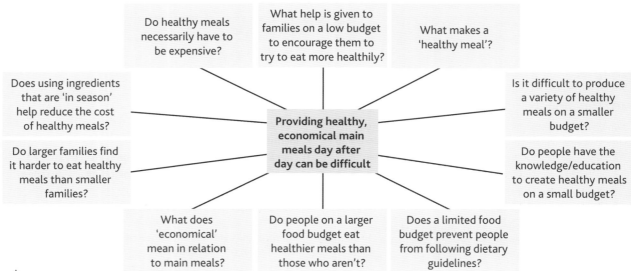

A Example of a GCSE student's task analysis

Evaluation

You will need to evaluate both your Individual Investigation and also the Research Task part of your Controlled Assessment. This should include a discussion of the following:

1 What you set out to do in your task analysis.
2 The conclusions drawn from your research.
3 The aims identified and whether they were achieved.
4 The practical solutions planned.
5 Results of the practical activities.
6 Sensory and nutritional analysis.
7 Conclusions drawn and what you have learned from doing this investigation.

B *Assessment objectives for the Individual Investigation*

Outline of content	Suggested class time	Assessment objective tested
Task analysis to include: • nutritional needs of teenagers • economical ingredients • skills and time needed to cook dishes.	2 hours	AO1
Carry out research including a survey or questionnaire on the target group, to establish: • likes and dislikes • food preparation skills • time, money and equipment available for food preparation and cooking.	2 hours	AO1
• Analyse the information collected. • Draw conclusions. • Produce a statement of aims for planning the practical solution.	2 hours	AO2
• Plan your practical work with justification for your choice of dishes. • Make sure you produce time plans, recipes and methods, with details of sensory testing you might do.	2 hours	AO2
• Make the planned dishes in the practical lessons and carry out taste tests on some of the dishes made. • Remember to photograph your finished work to put into your finished investigation.	6 hours	AO2
• Evaluate the practical dishes made. Using your sensory analysis charts, comment on the appearance, taste and texture of your finished dishes.	1 hour	AO3
• Carry out nutritional analysis of the dishes made and compare the results with your research on the nutritional needs of teenagers.	1 hour	
• Work out the cost of each dish and the cost per portion, and comment on which dishes were most economical.	1 hour	
• Review all aspects of the investigation, and draw conclusions on the solution you produced for the task set.	1 hour	AO3

Tuna Pasta Bake

This dish also uses a cheese sauce which provides HBV protein, vitamins A, B and D and calcium. The tuna provides HBV protein, vitamins A, B and D and some fat which is needed in the diet in small amounts. I used tinned tuna which is cheaper than fresh and has a long shelf life. The pasta bulks the dish out as it is a filling staple food. It is also very cheap and quick to cook (it takes between 12 and 15 minutes depending on the type of pasta used).

I used white pasta although wholewheat is a healthier choice and helps you to feel full for longer. The peas and sweetcorn added colour and because they were frozen required no preparation time, making it more economical for time. You could also use other vegetables such as green beans to add variety. This dish is healthy because it includes the right proportions of the various food groups seen on the eatwell plate.

The dish was quick to make and the melted cheese made it look more attractive once it had been cooked, and gave the pasta directly underneath a crispy texture. This dish could be served with either vegetables or salad.

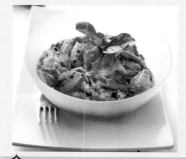

C *Example of a GCSE student's evaluation of practical work*

6.3 Research Task

What will I have to do for the Research Task?

1 Choose a topic from a range of tasks provided by AQA.
2 Collect background information on the topic.
3 Analyse the information and identify the problem for investigation.
4 Plan a practical solution relating to the research findings.
5 Carry out the practical work including sensory testing where appropriate.
6 Evaluate your investigation in the form of a written report on the outcomes.

Objectives

Understand how to carry out the Research Task part of your Controlled Assessment.

A *Example of a Research Task*

Outline of content	Suggested class time	Assessment objective tested
Background information on the main different cultural influences on the choice of food.	1 hour	AO1
Shopping survey of food from different cultures.	1–2 hours	AO1 and AO2
Focusing on one of the cultures researched: • select and make a typical dish • carry out a comparative analysis with a ready made equivalent.	1 hour planning 2 hours comparative analysis	AO2
Evaluate your investigation and produce a written report on the outcomes.	1–2 hours	AO3

Investigation 🔍

Example of a Research Task

Investigate the ways in which cultural diversity affects the food choices we make.

Guidelines for the written report

1 List the main points of the information which you collected about the different cultural influences on our choice of food.
2 Describe the research methods used and say which gave you the most useful information.
3 Discuss which culture you focused on, and justify your choice.
4 Describe the practical work you did and evaluate the end results.
5 Describe the **comparative analysis** of a home made dish with a ready made equivalent, and draw **conclusions** on your results.
6 Evaluate all the work you have done, identify the strengths and weaknesses of your investigation, and suggest improvements that might be made.

Key terms

Comparative analysis: looking at the characteristics of two or more products of a similar kind.

Conclusions: drawing together information and extracting the main points.

How to carry out a sensory analysis

Sensory analysis, or taste testing, helps you to draw conclusions from your practical work. This is also a useful process to use in your Individual Investigation (see 6.2). For more information on sensory analysis, see 2.3.

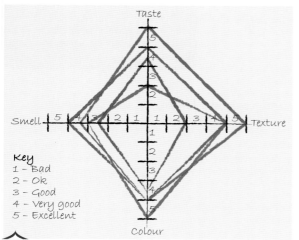

Key
1 – Bad
2 – Ok
3 – Good
4 – Very good
5 – Excellent

Taster	Taste	Texture	Colour	Smell
A	5	5	4	3.5
B	4	4	4	4
C	3.5	2	3.5	2.5
D	2	4	5	3

B Example of a GCSE student's sensory analysis using a star profile

How to carry out a nutritional analysis

Once you have finished your practical work, you need to carry out a nutritional analysis of the dishes made so that you can discuss whether you have produced a nutritionally balanced dish. This is also useful for your Individual Investigation. You can use a nutritional analysis program to do this and present your results as a graph, but you should also discuss the results and relate them to the criteria set in the task. See Diagram **C** for an example of a nutritional analysis graph with comments. For more information on nutritional analysis using computer programs, see 1.3.

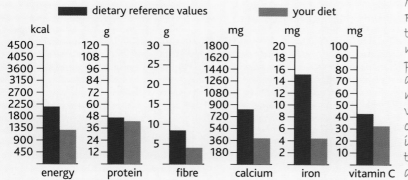

Nutritional analysis of Mushroom, Bacon and Cheese Risotto

■ dietary reference values   ■ your diet

Mushroom, Bacon and Cheese Risotto would serve between three and four people and the nutritional analysis shows that it provides a high amount of energy and is a good source of protein. To maximise the amount of iron and vitamin C in this meal, the risotto could be served with a salad. Iron is needed to help build blood in the body and vitamin C helps the absorption of calcium.

Calcium could be increased by drinking milk with this meal; calcium is needed to help with the growth and maintenance of bones and teeth. This dish would help towards eating the recommended amount of fibre, although the amount of fibre provided by the risotto could be improved by using wholegrain rice instead of white rice.

C Example of a GCSE student's nutritional analysis

6.4 Primary research methods

What is primary research?

This is research where you collect the information yourself using different methods of **data** collection. These include questionnaires, surveys, case studies, dietary diaries, and interviews.

Objectives

Understand how to carry out primary research for both the Individual Investigation and the Research Task.

Questionnaires

Pilot Questionnaire

Aim: to find out whether people are eating healthy economical meals.

1. How many people do you live with? (Please tick appropriate box)

   1 ☐   3 ☐   5 ☐   7 ☐
   2 ☐   4 ☐   6 ☐   8+ ☐

2a. Do you have any children?

   Yes ☐
   No ☐

2b. If yes, what are their ages?

3. What is your occupation?

4. What bracket does your weekly food budget fall into? (Please tick appropriate box)
   £0–£40   ☐
   £40–£80   ☐
   £80–£120   ☐
   £120–£160   ☐
   £160+   ☐

5a. Do you think your diet is healthy?
   Yes ☐
   No ☐

5b. What do you think makes a healthy diet?

6a. Do you eat the recommended 5 portions of fruit and vegetables a day?
   Yes ☐
   No ☐

6b. If no, why not?

7. Do you regularly buy foods that are in season?
   Yes ☐
   No ☐

A *Example of a GCSE student's pilot questionnaire*

Justifications for Pilot Questionnaire

By doing a questionnaire my aim was to find out whether people (and in particular families) are eating healthy main meals and how much they spend on food. I asked specific questions that I hoped would help me in my investigation.

1. I asked how many people they lived with so I could understand whether they were providing meals for a small or large family.

2. I asked whether they had children because I thought people with young children were more likely to eat healthily.

3. By asking what their occupation was I wanted to get an idea of what income they had without actually asking them.

4. By asking what bracket their food budget fell into I wanted to know whether they were on a limited food budget.

5. I asked whether they thought their diet to be healthy because I wanted to find out if their budget affected their diet. I then asked what they thought made a healthy diet to check they knew what one was.

6. I asked whether they ate 5 portions of fruit and vegetables a day, and asked why not if they didn't, to find out what their reason was, e.g. the price of fruit or vegetables may affect their intake.

7. I asked whether they bought fruit and vegetables that are in season often as it makes them cheaper and they are generally of better quality.

B *Justifications for pilot questionnaire*

A questionnaire is a useful way of finding out information about a topic from a group of people. To carry out a questionnaire you need to follow these steps:

1 Identify the **target group**: for example, you might want to find out what Year 10 students think about school dinners.

2 Decide how many people will be in the **sample group**: for example, 10 boys and 10 girls.

3 Decide what you want to find out: for example, which foods are most popular or how often a person eats school meals.

4 Keep the questions easy to understand and do not have too many, so that they can be answered fairly quickly.

5 Decide on a time and place to carry out your questionnaire and make a note of this in your planning.

6 You might want to test your questionnaire with a **pilot** that you carry out on a few people. This is to see if there are any problems with the questions before you do the final questionnaire.

7 Conduct your questionnaire.

8 Present the results of your questionnaire in the form of a bar or pie chart. Use a computer program to draw the charts, if possible.

9 Write a summary of the results from each question.

10 Draw conclusions from the information gathered.

> ## Key terms
>
> **Data**: an item of information.
>
> **Target group**: the type of people you are investigating: for example, teenagers.
>
> **Sample group**: those people within the target group who you ask to complete your questionnaire: the people in your class, for example.
>
> **Pilot**: a test on a small sample that you carry out before conducting the actual questionnaire.

> ## AQA Examiner's tip
>
> When planning questionnaires, vary the questions asked so that some are 'open' questions with several possible answers, and some are 'closed' questions where the answers are either yes or no.

Final Questionnaire Results

Q1 How many people live in your house?

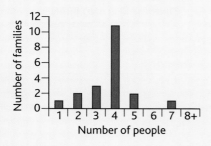

Although I wanted to get a variety of different sized households to complete my questionnaire, I wanted to concentrate on families in particular because that's what my hypothesis is focused on. I achieved this as the majority of those completing my questionnaire lived with more than one person. Eleven people were part of a family of four, which is a common number to have in a family.

Q2 What are the occupations of the adults in your household?

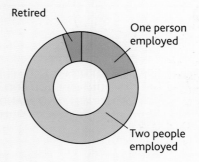

Most households had two people in employment which suggests that the majority were not on a limited budget, although some worked part-time. No-one was unemployed and so relying on government benefits.

 Example of a GCSE student's questionnaire results

Surveys

A survey is similar to a questionnaire except that you observe and record the information for yourself. For example, you might want to investigate the range of multicultural foods available in different shops. To do this, you would have to get permission from the shop manager by phoning or writing a letter.

Case studies

These are useful if you are collecting information on special dietary needs, such as diabetes or coronary heart disease. You will need to visit someone with the condition to find out as much information as possible about how the condition affects their life. This is a useful research method if you already know someone with a special dietary need.

Dietary diaries

These are a record of all the food and drink that a person consumes over a given period. The information collected can then be analysed using a nutritional analysis program and nutrient deficiencies can be identified. (See 1.3).

Monday Day 2   Date......................

BEFORE BREAKFAST	
TIME	AMOUNT OF FOOD AND DRINK TAKEN AND BRAND
7.00 am	apple juice (small glass)

BREAKFAST	
TIME	AMOUNT OF FOOD AND DRINK TAKEN AND BRAND
8.00 am	1 medium bowl cornflakes with semi-skimmed milk 1 large banana

MID-MORNING BETWEEN BREAKFAST AND MIDDAY MEAL	
TIME	AMOUNT OF FOOD AND DRINK TAKEN AND BRAND
11.00 pm	Kit kat (2 fingers) bag of crisps (Walkers) small carton of apple juice

MIDDAY MEAL	
TIME	AMOUNT OF FOOD AND DRINK TAKEN AND BRAND
12.30 pm	School pizza, chips and baked beans Chocolate muffin (medium) Small glass water

EVENING MEAL	
TIME	AMOUNT OF FOOD AND DRINK TAKEN AND BRAND
6.00 pm	Small portion spaghetti bolognese (home-made) Medium apple

D *Example of a GCSE student's dietary diary*

Interviews

These are usually carried out with a person who has specialist knowledge of the topic you are investigating. For example, a dietician can be interviewed for advice on dietary diseases; a dentist about the effect of sugar on teeth; or the catering manager for information on school meals. You need to prepare a list of questions before you carry out an interview, so that you can cover all the information required for your investigation.

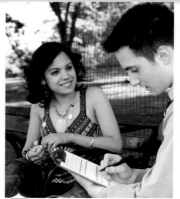

E *Student carrying out a survey*

6.5 Secondary research methods

What is secondary research?

Secondary research is information you collect that someone else has produced. You can find this information in books, leaflets, magazines, newspaper articles or websites.

Books

When researching topics from books, use several and compare the information given. Use content pages and **indexes** to find the information you need. Pick out the key points from each book, and summarise in your own words what you have learned about the topic. Do not copy out chunks of the book as you will not receive any marks for copying. You can **quote** small sections to illustrate a point you are making, but you must put quotes in inverted commas and give the **book reference**.

Websites

Only use valid websites such as those quoted in this book. Treat information from websites in the same way as that from books, and remember that you will not gain any marks for just including masses of printouts. You will only gain credit for information you have discussed.

Objectives

Understand how to carry out secondary research for both the Individual Investigation and the Research Task.

Present your investigation.

Key terms

Index: an alphabetical list of topics, usually at the end of a book.

Quote: copy of an extract from a book or website, in quotation marks, with the source acknowledged.

Book reference: when using a quote, give the book title, author and page number.

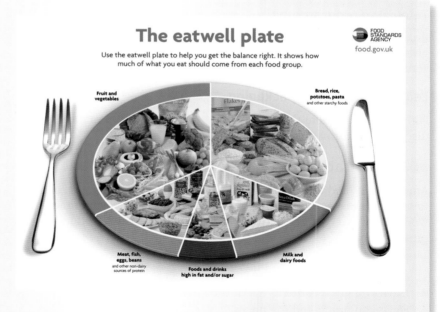

The eatwell plate has been produced in the UK by the Food Standards Agency to show that a healthy balanced diet contains a variety of types of food, including lots of fruit, vegetables and starchy foods, some protein-rich foods, and some dairy foods. Similarly, in the USA a food guide pyramid has been developed to help people with daily food choices.

The largest segment on the eatwell plate is starchy foods. Starchy food should make up about a third of the food you eat, as should fruits and vegetables. Studies have shown that most people should be eating more starchy foods. Starchy foods are made from cereal crops (such as wheat, barley and corn) and are a good source of energy (they are high in carbohydrates which provides the body with energy) and the main source of a range of nutrients in our diet.

The eatwell plate

Use the eatwell plate to help you get the balance right. It shows how much of what you eat should come from each food group.

FOOD STANDARDS AGENCY
food.gov.uk

Fruit and vegetables

Bread, rice, potatoes, pasta and other starchy foods

Meat, fish, eggs, beans and other non-dairy sources of protein

Foods and drinks high in fat and/or sugar

Milk and dairy foods

 A *Example of a GCSE student using material from a government website*

Newspaper and magazine articles

You may include photocopies of relevant articles but, if they are large, try to reduce them so that they do not take up too much space. Always give your own viewpoint on the articles included, or write your own version of the report, as in the example provided in Diagram **B**.

Articles in the Media related to my Investigation

I have gathered evidence from newspapers and the internet that are relevant to my investigation. These articles have answered many of the questions I asked myself in my analysis of my investigation title at the beginning of my investigation. I have summarised what each article has told me, how this relates to my investigation and whether it supports or goes against my hypothesis.

The Telegraph Newspaper

This article is about research that suggests that people on a low-income are not the only ones with a poor diet and that they have virtually the same level of nutrition as the general population. It also says that the majority of people belonging to a low-income family can cook meals from basic ingredients which suggests that knowledge is not one of the main reasons why such families struggle to produce main meals. Overall this article goes against my hypothesis that it is more difficult for families to produce healthy main meals and instead suggests that the population as a whole are struggling to eat a balanced diet. This article also suggests that the link between a poor diet and a low-income is not as strong as people may think.

B Example of a GCSE student's viewpoint on newspaper articles used in their research

Television programmes

If you are using a TV programme for your research, make sure you give the date and the content of the programme, and discuss how it contributes to your research.

Leaflets, labels and packaging

Only use these where they are relevant to the topic, and make sure you discuss the information provided by them.

Presentation of your Controlled Assessment

After all your hard work, make sure you present your Investigation and Research Task as neatly as possible, including photos of all your practical work. Below is a checklist for what you should make sure to include in your presentation.

- Front page should have: the title of the investigation; your name and candidate number; the centre number.
- Have you got a contents list at the beginning?
- Have you numbered the pages?
- Have you labelled all diagrams and photographs?
- You do not need to put each page into individual plastic wallets, but your work does need to be held together in a soft folder.
- If your work is handwritten, is it easy to read?
- Make sure you check your spellings, punctuation and grammar.
- Headings and separate paragraphs help to make your written work easier to read.
- Is there a bibliography and a list of references?

Remember

Use a variety of primary and secondary research methods in your Investigation and Research Task.

Bibliography

Books used in my coursework:

- *Food and Nutrition* by Anita Tull
- *Examining Food and Nutrition* by Jenny Ridgwell
- *Feasts for a Fiver* by Sophie Grigson
- *Human Nutrition* by Mary E. Barasi

Websites used in my coursework:

- www.bbc.co.uk
- www.food.gov.uk
- www.eatwell.gov.uk
- www.bbcgoodfood.com
- www.wikipedia.com
- www.answers.com
- www.irf.org.uk
- www.telegraph.co.uk
- www.keighleynews.co.uk

C Example of a GCSE student's bibliography

AQA Examination-style questions

1 Nutrition, diet and health

1 (a) Which **three** nutrients supply the body with energy? *(3 marks)*
(b) Explain what happens if we eat more food than our body requires. *(2 marks)*
(c) Why do energy needs change with age? *(2 marks)*

AQA 2007

2 (a) Name **three** good sources of plant protein foods. *(3 marks)*
(b) Explain, with an example, the complementary action of proteins. *(2 marks)*

AQA specimen paper

3 What is meant by:
(a) a balanced diet?
(b) malnutrition?
(c) basal metabolic rate? *(6 marks)*

AQA 2007

4 (a) What are the functions of calcium in the diet? *(2 marks)*
(b) Name the vitamin needed for the proper absorption of calcium. *(1 mark)*

AQA 2007

5 (a) Why is it important to include dietary fibre (NSP) in the diet? *(2 marks)*
(b) Name **two** foods which are a good source of dietary fibre. *(2 marks)*
(c) Name **two** health conditions which may be caused by low dietary fibre intake. *(2 marks)*

AQA specimen paper

6 (a) Give **three** reasons why a person may become a vegetarian. *(3 marks)*
(b) Name **two** foods that are rich in iron and suitable for a vegetarian. *(2 marks)*

AQA specimen paper

7 The Guideline Daily Amounts (GDA) for adults are shown below.

	GDA Women	GDA Men
Energy – kcal (calories)	2000	2500
Fat	70 g	90 g
of which are saturates	20 g	30 g
Salt	6 g	6 g

(a) How do these guidelines help us to make healthy choices? *(2 marks)*
(b) Explain why men and women have different nutritional requirements. *(2 marks)*

AQA 2008

8   Guidelines for healthy eating are shown below.

Base your meals on starch   Eat lots of fruit and vegetables
Eat more fish   Cut down on saturated fat
Cut down on sugar   Try to eat less salt
Drink plenty of water   Don't skip breakfast

Discuss how each of these guidelines can improve health. Give practical examples
of each guideline.   *(15 marks)*

AQA 2008

9   What are the functions of enzymes in the digestive system?   *(2 marks)*

AQA 2006

10   Copy and complete the table below to show the enzyme involved in digestion and
the substance produced.

Nutrient	Enzyme	Simpler substance produced
Protein		
Fats		
Starch		

(6 marks)

AQA 2006

2   Nutritional, physical, chemical and sensory properties of food

1   Explain what happens if vegetables are left to soak in water before cooking.   *(2 marks)*

AQA 2007

2   What happens to cheese when it is cooked?   *(2 marks)*

AQA 2007

3   Margarine is fortified with **two** vitamins. Which vitamins are these?   *(2 marks)*

AQA 2005

4   Describe the changes that take place during the cooking of white sauce.   *(6 marks)*

AQA 2007

5   What is the effect of dry heat on starch?   *(2 marks)*

AQA 2006

6   How can the loss of water soluble vitamins be prevented when preparing and
cooking vegetables?   *(4 marks)*

AQA 2008

7   Which nutrients are added to white flour when it is fortified?   *(3 marks)*

AQA 2008

8   The method of cooking can affect the nutritional value of foods.
Compare the nutritional values of:
  (a)   roast potatoes and baked jacket potatoes   *(2 marks)*
  (b)   steamed broccoli and boiled broccoli   *(2 marks)*

AQA 2006

9   Describe the physical and chemical changes that take place when boiling an egg.   *(6 marks)*

AQA 2003

10   Vegetables can be cooked in a variety of ways. State **one** advantage and **one** disadvantage of each of the following:

   (a)   Boiling vegetables
      (i)   Advantage
      (ii)   Disadvantage   *(2 marks)*
   (b)   Roasting vegetables
      (i)   Advantage
      (ii)   Disadvantage   *(2 marks)*
   (c)   Grilling vegetables
      (i)   Advantage
      (ii)   Disadvantage   *(2 marks)*

AQA 2003

(3) Techniques and skills in food storage, preparation and cooking

1   Copy the table below and complete the empty boxes to show how you would store foods in the home.

Type of food	Recommended storage	Example of food
Perishable		
Frozen		

(4 marks)

AQA 2008

2   Give **three** reasons for cooking food.   *(3 marks)*

AQA specimen paper

3   Explain the meaning of the following terms:
   (a)   Conduction
   (b)   Convection
   (c)   Radiation   *(6 marks)*

AQA specimen paper

4   List **five** pieces of electrical equipment you could buy to save time and effort when preparing and cooking food.   *(5 marks)*

AQA 2007

5   Give **one** advantage and **one** disadvantage of fruit in the following forms:
   (a)   Fresh fruit
   (b)   Frozen fruit
   (c)   Canned fruit
   (d)   Dried fruit   *(8 marks)*

AQA 2007

6   Give **three** attachments you might find on a food processor. For each attachment give an example of how it could be used.

For example: Attachment:
   Use:

(6 marks)

AQA 2008

7   Peas can be bought fresh, frozen, dried and canned. Compare the nutritional value of these types of peas.

(4 marks)

AQA 2008

8   Discuss the advantages and disadvantages of microwave cooking.

(8 marks)

AQA 2003

9   Give **three** ways air can be added to a mixture.

(3 marks)

AQA 2007

10 Explain why the following additives are used in food products:
   (a) Preservatives
   (b) Antioxidants
   (c) Colourings
   (d) Emulsifiers
   (e) Flavourings

(5 marks)

AQA 2001

4   Factors affecting consumer choice

1   List **five** points to consider before planning an evening meal for a family.

(5 marks)

AQA 2007

2   Nutritional needs vary at different life stages. Discuss the nutritional needs during pregnancy and for the elderly. Give examples of how these needs can be met.

(12 marks)

AQA 2007

3   Some elderly people live alone. Describe some of the problems which could affect their diet.

(9 marks)

AQA 2008

4   Give **three** guidelines to help an elderly person spend their money wisely in the supermarket.

(3 marks)

AQA 2008

5   What is the purpose of the Trades Descriptions Act?

(2 marks)

AQA 2006

6   State **two** Consumer rights under the Sale and Supply of Goods Act.

(2 marks)

AQA 2003

7   State **two** aims of the Food Safety Act of 1990.

(2 marks)

AQA 2003

8   Many children eat snacks between meals. Give **three** examples of healthy snack foods.

(3 marks)

AQA 2007

9   Explain the factors you should consider when choosing a new cooker.

(9 marks)

AQA 2006

10 (a) What are the advantages of shopping for food in a supermarket?   *(4 marks)*
(b) What are the advantages and disadvantages of shopping for food on the internet?   *(6 marks)*

AQA 2007

5 Food hygiene and safety

1 What advice would you give for the safe storage of food in a refrigerator?   *(4 marks)*

AQA 2007

2 Explain the following abbreviations/ terms:
(a) AFD
(b) MAP
(c) Cook-chill   *(6 marks)*

AQA 2008

3 Explain the effects of temperature control on food safety.   *(4 marks)*

AQA 2008

4 (a) List **two** common symptoms of food poisoning.   *(2 marks)*
(b) Name **three** bacteria which may cause food poisoning.   *(3 marks)*
(c) Give **two** examples of high risk foods which could cause food poisoning.   *(2 marks)*

AQA specimen paper

5 Complete the following sentences to show how bacteria are controlled by temperature.
(a) The temperature of a home freezer should be __ °C
(b) Food in a refrigerator should be stored below __ °C
(c) Cooked food should be heated to at least __°C at its centre   *(3 marks)*

AQA specimen paper

6 List **six** pieces of information which must, by law, be shown on a food label.   *(6 marks)*

AQA 2008

7 (a) Explain the difference between 'use by' and 'best before' dates on food packaging.   *(2 marks)*
(b) What is meant by shelf life?   *(1 mark)*

AQA 2008

8 Why are some foods packaged before they are sold?   *(4 marks)*

AQA 2006

9 Give **three** modern developments in food packaging.   *(3 marks)*

AQA 2006

10 Read the newspaper report below.

> A butcher was selling raw and cooked meats in his shop. In one week in June, 50 of his customers became ill with salmonella food poisoning.
>
> After investigation it was found that the butcher had used the same wooden chopping board for slicing both the raw and the cooked meats.
>
> Tests on the refrigerator found the temperature to be 10°C.

(a) Give **two** reasons why people who bought meat from this shop suffered from salmonella food poisoning.   *(2 marks)*
(b) What precautions should the butcher have taken to prevent this?   *(2 marks)*

AQA 2008

Glossary

A

accelerated freeze drying (AFD): method of food preservation where food is frozen first before the ice crystals are removed in a vacuum.

aerobic bacteria: bacteria which need oxygen to grow.

ageing population: a population where there are more elderly people than young people.

allergic: see allergy.

allergy: where the body reacts adversely to certain foods.

amino acids: chemicals which make up protein molecules.

amylase: digestive enzyme that breaks down carbohydrates.

anaerobic bacteria: bacteria which do not need oxygen to grow.

anaphylactic shock: severe symptom of food allergy, where sufferer has difficulty breathing.

antibacterial: prevents bacteria from spreading.

appetising: looks and smells good to eat.

B

bacteria: single-celled organisms which occur naturally in soil, air, water, and on humans and animals; some can be harmful to humans.

balanced diet: a diet that contains all the nutrients in the correct amounts to meet individual needs.

basal metabolic rate (BMR): the rate at which the body uses energy when it is warm and resting.

beta-carotene: form of vitamin A found in vegetable sources.

blanch: cooking vegetables or fruit in boiling water for short periods to inactivate enzymes which may cause deterioration.

blind tastings: consumer tests on new food products, where the tester does not know which food they are tasting.

book reference: when using a quote, give the book title, author and page number.

C

calcium: mineral needed for strong bones and teeth.

calorie (kilocalories or kcal): unit of energy provided by food.

capacity: storage size of fridges and freezers in litres.

caramelisation: browning of sugar when dry heat is applied.

carbohydrates: the cheapest and healthiest source of energy in our diets.

cholesterol: fatty substance that can cause blockages in the arteries.

coagulation: setting of proteins during heating.

coeliac disease: a condition where sufferers are sensitive to gluten in wheat and other cereal products.

comparative analysis: looking at the characteristics of two or more products of a similar kind.

complementation of protein: eating different vegetable protein foods together in order to ensure intake of all the essential amino acids.

component: a discrete assessable element within a controlled assessment/qualification that is not itself formally reported, where the marks are recorded by the awarding body. A component/unit may contain one or more tasks.

conclusions: drawing together information and extracting the main points.

conduction: heat conducted through molecules in solids and liquids.

consumer protection: laws to make sure that the goods and services you buy are of a satisfactory quality and fit for purpose.

controlled assessment: a form of internal assessment where the control levels are set for each stage of the assessment process: task setting; task taking; and task marking.

convection: heat moving through liquids and gases by convection currents.

cook-chill: foods which have been partly or fully cooked and then chilled by the manufacturer.

coronary heart disease (CHD): condition where blood flow to the heart is reduced because of a build up of a fatty substance in the arteries which lead to the heart.

D

data: an item of information.

denaturation: change in chemical structure of proteins during heating.

dextrinisation: browning of starches when dry heat is applied.

diabetes: condition where there is too much glucose in the blood because the body cannot use it properly.

dietary diary: a record of all the food and drink intake of a person over a given period of days.

dietary fibre: refers to non-starch polysaccharides which are found in fruit and vegetables.

dietary reference value (DRV): overall term used to cover EAR, LRNI and RNI.

digestion: process of food being broken down in the body so that the nutrients can be absorbed.

digestive enzymes: chemicals in the digestive juices which speed up the breakdown of food and the release of nutrients.

disposable income: money left after tax and other deductions have been made from a persons earnings.

dry methods: cooking with no added liquid but fat sometimes used to prevent food sticking to tins.

E

E coli: type of bacteria which can cause food poisoning.

E numbers: additives approved by the European Union.

efficient: performing a task without wasting time and energy.

emulsifiers: additives used to mix water and oil together in a stable solution and to prevent separation.

energy balance: when the energy intake of food equals that used up in energy expenditure.

energy dense: containing high amounts of fat and sugar.

energy rating: how much energy an appliance uses: energy consumption, kWh/year.

energy saving: using less power, such as electricity or gas.

enzymes: molecules in foods which cause ripening or change the structure.

essential amino acids: indispensable amino acids which we cannot live without and which must be obtained from the diet.

estimated average requirement (EAR): average amount of a given nutrient required by a group of people.

external assessment: a form of independent assessment in which question papers, assignments and tasks are set by the awarding body, taken under specified conditions (including detailed supervision and duration) and marked by the awarding body.

extractives: savoury flavours that develop in meat as it cooks.

extrinsic sugars (added sugars): sugars which are not part of the cell structure of plants, but are added to foods to provide sweetness and a quick source of energy.

F

fat-soluble vitamins: vitamins A, D, E and K which are present in the fat content of foods.

food additive: natural or chemical substance added to food to improve quality.

food miles: the distance food has travelled from harvesting, processing and packaging before it reaches the consumer.

food poisoning: a common illness that is caused by eating foods that are contaminated with harmful bacteria.

fortified: where nutrients are added to improve the nutritional value of a product.

G

GDA (guideline daily amounts): guidelines based on DRVs which have been developed by food manufactures and retailers to simplify nutritional information on food labels.

gelatinisation: thickening of starch when moist heat is applied.

glucose: the simple sugar which carbohydrates are broken down into before being absorbed into the bloodstream.

glycemic index (GI): the rate at which carbohydrates are converted into glucose during digestion.

grazing: snacking throughout the day.

guideline daily amounts: see GDA.

H

haem iron: type of iron which is found in meat and is easily absorbed by the body.

haemoglobin: component of red blood cells which contains iron and is needed for carrying oxygen in the bloodstream.

heat transfer: the process by which heat energy is transferred to food.

high biological value (HBV) proteins: proteins from animal sources which contain all of the indispensable (essential) amino acids.

high risk foods: foods which are easily contaminated with food poisoning bacteria.

hydrogenation: process of hardening fats to make margarine which makes the fat more saturated.

I

incubation period: the time between eating infected food and becoming ill with food poisoning.

index: an alphabetical list of topics, usually at the end of a book.

indispensable amino acids: essential amino acids which we can not live without.

individual nutritional requirements: the amount of nutrients needed to maintain good health based on age, gender, physical activity and state of health.

insulin: hormone made in the pancreas which controls transport of glucose into the body's cells.

intrinsic sugars (sometimes called natural sugars): form part of the cell structure of plants in some fruits and vegetables.

iron: mineral needed for healthy red blood cells and carrying oxygen round the body.

irradiation: treatment of food with radiation to kill micro-organisms.

L

labour saving: saving effort by the cook.

lacto-ovo-vegetarian: vegetarian who will eat dairy products and eggs, but not meat, poultry or fish.

lactose: intrinsic (natural) sugar found in milk and milk products.

lacto-vegetarian: vegetarian who does not eat meat, poultry, fish or eggs; but will eat dairy products.

lecithin: chemical in egg yolk which acts as an emulsifying agent.

lipase: digestive enzyme that breaks down fats.

low biological value (LBV) proteins: proteins from vegetable proteins sources which lack one or more of the indispensable (essential) amino acids.

lower reference nutrient intake (LRNI): the amount of nutrient that is enough for a few people in a population group who have low needs.

M

malnutrition: lack of food or particular nutrients in the diet or too much of the wrong kinds of food, causing obesity.

mark scheme a scheme detailing how credit is to be awarded in relation to a particular unit, component or task. A mark scheme normally characterises acceptable answers or levels of response to questions/tasks or parts of questions/tasks and identifies the amount of credit each attracts.

media: TV, radio, newspapers, magazines and the internet.

micronutrients: vitamins and minerals.

micro-organisms: yeasts, moulds and bacteria.

minerals: micronutrients needed in small amounts in the diet but having many important functions in the body.

modified atmosphere packaging (MAP): method of packaging food products where oxygen is removed from the packaging and replaced with an inert gas such as carbon dioxide or nitrogen; this slows down food spoilage and the development of micro-organisms.

modify: alter recipes to reduce fat, salt or sugar, or increase fibre.

moist methods: cooking with added liquid.

monosodium glutamate: additive used to enhance flavour of foods.

N

non-haem iron: type of iron which is obtained from non-meat sources and is less easily absorbed by the body than haem iron.

non-perishable: foods which have been processed to prevent rapid decay.

non-starch polysaccharide (NSP) (also known as dietary fibre): the indigestible fibrous structure of plants; it is not a nutrient, but is essential for the elimination of waste products from the large intestine.

novel foods: foods which are manufactured from ingredients not usually used for food.

novel proteins: proteins grown from micro-organisms which produce mycoproteins.

nutrients: chemical compounds found in foods, which include proteins, fats, carbohydrates, vitamins and minerals.

nutrition: the study of the nutrients found in food and their functions in the body.

nutritional supplements: additives used to improve the nutritional value of foods.

O

organic: foods that have been grown or reared without chemicals.

organised: using good working practice.

organoleptic: sensory qualities of food.

oxidation: exposure to air causing loss of vitamin C in fruits and vegetables.

P

partly processed: foods which have had some of the preparation done.

pathogenic bacteria: bacteria which are harmful to humans and can cause food poisoning.

peer group pressure: conforming to what friends choose.

pepsin: digestive enzyme which begins digestion of proteins in the stomach.

perishable: fresh foods which decay rapidly.

permitted additives: additives tested by the Food Standards Agency before being approved for use by food manufacturers.

pester power: children pestering adults to buy products.

physical activity level (PAL): an individual's level of activity which depends on their job and leisure activities.

pilot: a test on a small sample that you carry out before conducting a full investigation.

preservation: treatment of food to prevent decay and keep it safe to eat for longer periods than it would be in its natural state.

primary research: information that you find out for yourself.

product placement: putting products in prominent places, such as at the end of aisles or at the checkout.

proteins: building blocks of all body cells.

protein sparing: eating carbohydrates with proteins allowing the proteins to be used for growth and repair rather than for energy.

proteinase: digestive enzyme that breaks down proteins.

Q

quote: copy of an extract from a book or website, in quotation marks, with the source acknowledged.

R

radiation: infra-red rays directed onto food.

raising agents: products such as yeast and baking powder that produce gas when heated and so help flour mixtures to rise during cooking.

rancidity: unpleasant flavours which develop in fats when they are exposed to oxygen.

ready to eat: foods which can be consumed with no more cooking.

redress: remedy, rectify or put right.

reference nutrient intake (RNI): an amount of a nutrient that is enough, or more than enough, for approximately 97 per cent of a population group.

respiration: process in which air passes into and out of the lungs so that the blood can absorb oxygen and give off carbon dioxide and water.

S

salivary amylase: digestive enzyme in saliva which begins digestion of starch into sugars.

sample group: a small group of people within a target group who take part in your investigation.

saturated fats: fats from animal sources such as meat, eggs, milk, butter and cheese.

saturated fatty acids: have no double bonds, as all the carbon atoms are saturated with hydrogen.

secondary research: information that someone else has produced: for example, books, leaflets, magazines, newspaper articles and websites.

sensory analysis: a process carried out to analyse a food product using the senses of sight, smell, taste and hearing.

sensory testing: commenting on appearance, taste and texture.

slow releasing carbohydrates: foods which are converted to glucose slowly and provide energy over a relatively long period of time.

social groups: friends or members of clubs, churches or organisations to which a person belongs.

stabilisers: additives used to prevent separation of mixtures.

starchy foods: cereals, vegetables, fruit, pasta, rice, potatoes and bread.

statutory information: information which must be provided by law.

statutory regulations: Acts of parliament on which consumer law is based.

sterilisation: a heating process which kills bacteria.

stock rotation: checking best before dates on dry goods and using the oldest first.

T

tamper-proof seals: plastic collars on lids and shrink-wrapped jars to ensure that foods have not been contaminated.

target group: the type of people you are investigating.

task: a discrete element of external or controlled assessment that may include examinations, assignments, practical activities and projects.

task marking: this specifies the way in which credit is awarded for candidates' outcomes. Marking involves the use of mark schemes and/or marking criteria produced by the awarding body.

task setting: the specification of the assessment requirements. Tasks may be set by awarding bodies and/or teachers, as defined by subject-specific rules. Teacher-set tasks must be developed in line with awarding body specified requirements.

task taking: the conditions for candidate support and supervision, and the authentication of candidates' work. Task taking may involve different parameters from those used in traditional written examinations, for example, candidates may be allowed supervised access to sources such as the internet.

trace elements: minerals, including fluoride and iodine, which are needed in very small amounts in the diet.

traffic light labelling: a method of showing the fat, saturated fat, sugar and salt levels in foods using traffic light colours on the labels.

U

under-nutrition: eating too little for individual dietary needs.

unit: the smallest part of a qualification which is formally reported and can be separately certificated. A unit may comprise separately assessed components.

unsaturated fatty acids: fatty acids which have two or more double bonds.

V

vacuum packaging: plastic packaging where all the air has been removed.

vegan: vegetarian who will not eat any foods from animals, including milk and eggs, or use any products, such as cosmetics, shoes or clothes, which use animal products.

vitamins: micronutrients needed in the diet in small amounts and used by the body for protection from infection, and to regulate body processes such as the absorption of energy from food.

W

water soluble vitamins: vitamins B and C which dissolve in water.

weaning: the process of introducing solid foods into a baby's diet from six months old.

Y

yeasts: tiny, single-cell fungi which are found in the air and on the surface of some fruits; they are mostly harmless to humans.

Index

A

acids   14–17, 34–5
additives   38–9, 40–1
advertising   72–5
Advertising Standards Agency
   (ASA)   75
advice for consumers   73
aeration   54–5
aerobic bacteria   78
age   10–11, 62
ageing population   62
alkalis   34–5
allergies   64–5, 88
amino acids   14–15
anaerobic bacteria   78
anaphylactic shock   64–5
animal fats   16
animal protein   14–15
antibacterial cleaners   84
antioxidant vitamins   21
appearance of food   36
appetising food   41
ASA (Advertising Standards
   Agency)   75

B

babies   10–11
bacteria   78–81
balanced diet   8–9
basal metabolic rate
   (BMR)   26–7
bibliographies   100
blanching food   45
blenders   48, 71
blind tasting   36–7
BMR (basal metabolic
   rate)   26–7
book references   99
breastfeeding   10
browning   54

C

calcium   22–3
capacity   71
caramelisation   34–5
carbohydrates   18–19, 26–7
case studies   98
CHD (coronary heart disease)   66
chemical food properties   31–42
children's meals   65, 74
choice, consumers   59–76
cholesterol   66
chopping boards   47, 49
coagulation   34–5, 55
comparative analysis   94
complaints   74
conclusions   94–5
conduction   50–1
consumer choice   59–76
consumer protection   72–3
Controlled Assessment   91–100
   Individual Investigation   91–3
   objectives   91
   presentation   100
   primary research   92, 96–8
   Research Task   91, 93–5
   secondary research   92, 99–100
convection   50–1
convenience foods   56–7
cook-chill foods   56
cookers   48–9, 51, 64, 70
cooking food   33–7, 46–53
coronary heart disease (CHD)   66
coursework   91–100

D

data   96–8
deficiency   15
denaturation   34–5
dextrinisation   34
diabetics   66
diaries, dietary   12–13, 98

diet   7–30
dietary analysis   12–13
dietary diaries   12–13, 98
dietary fibre   18–19, 24
dietary reference value (DRV)   25,
   27
digestion   28–9
disposable income   62–3
DRV (dietary reference value)   25,
   27
dry cooking methods   52–3

E

E coli bacteria   80–1
E numbers   39
eating out   63
eatwell plate   9, 99
economic factors   62–3
efficiency   46
electrical equipment   49–50, 70–1
emulsifiers   54
energy   26–7, 49, 71
energy dense foods   26
energy rating   71
energy saving   49
enrichment   55
enzymes   28–9, 32–3
equipment   46–50, 70–1
examination-style questions   101–5
extractives   36–7

F

family background   60
family meals   64–5
family size   62–3
fat-soluble vitamins   20–1
fats   16–17
   energy   26–7
   food preparation   34
   saturated   16–17, 24, 66
   vitamins   20–1
fibre   18–19, 24

flavourings   54
Food Labelling Regulations
   1995   73
food miles   68–9
food mixers   48
food poisoning   79–81
food processors   48, 65, 71
food-related disorders   64–5
Food Safety Act 1990   72
fortification   40–1
freezers   70–1
fridges   70–1
frying methods   52

G

GDAs (guideline daily
   amounts)   25, 88–9
gelatinisation   34–5
gender   10–11
GI (glycemic index)   26
glossary   106–9
glycemic index (GI)   26
government nutrition
   guidelines   24–5
grazing   64–5
guideline daily amounts
   (GDAs)   25, 88–9

H

health   7–30
heart disease   66–7
heat transfer   50–1
high risk foods   82–3
hygiene and safety   77–90
   food poisoning   79–81
   procedures   82–5
   spoilage organisms   78–9

I

illness   11, 66–7
incubation periods   80–1
indexes   99
indispensable amino acids   14
Individual Investigation   91–3
individual nutritional
   requirements   10–11
information, nutrition   24–5

interviews   98
iron   22–3

K

knives   47, 49

L

labelling   88–9, 100
labour saving   49
leaflets   100
legislation   72–3
lifestyle change   60
liquidisers   48, 71

M

macronutrients   14–19
magazine articles   99
malnutrition   8–9
meal planning   64–7
media   64
metabolic rate   26–7
micronutrients   20–3
micro-organisms   78–9
microwave ovens   48–9, 51, 64,
   70
minerals   20–3
mixers   48, 71
modifying recipes   54–5
moist cooking methods   52–3
moulds   78

N

newspaper articles   99–100
non-perishable foods   44–5
non-starch polysaccharide
   (NSP)   18–19
novel food   40–1
novel proteins   14–15
NSP (non-starch
   polysaccharide)   18–19
nutrients   8–9
   digestion   28–9
   food storage   32–3
   macronutrients   14–19
   micronutrients   20–3
   preservation   85
nutrition   7–42, 95

O

organic foods   68–9
organisation   46
organoleptic food qualities   50
ovens   48–9, 51, 64, 70
oxidation   32–3

P

packaging   86–7, 100
PAL (physical activity level)
   10–11
partly processed foods   56
pathogenic bacteria   80–1
peer group pressure   60–1
perishable foods   44–5
permitted additives   39, 41
pester power   74
physical activity level (PAL)
   10–11
physical food properties   31–42
pilot tests   96–7
planning meals   64–7
poisoning   79–81
pregnancy   10–11, 65
preparation of food   34–7, 46–9
preservation   55, 84–5
primary research   92, 96–8
processed foods   56
processors   48, 64, 71
product placement   74
properties of food   31–42
proteins   14–15, 26–7, 34–5
purchasing food   68–9

Q

questionnaires   96–7
Quorn   15, 40
quotes   99

R

radiation   50–1
raising agents   55
rancidity   32–3
ready to eat foods   56
recipe balance   54–5
recycling   86

redress   73, 74
references   99
refridgerators   70–1
regulations   72–3
religious festivals   61
Research Task   91, 93–5
respiration   28–9
retail outlets   68–9

S

safe intake   25
safety   25, 71, 77–90
    see also hygiene and safety
Sale and Supply of Goods Act
    1994   72
saliva   28–9
sample groups   97
saturated fats   16–17, 24, 66
saturated fatty acids   16–17
scales   47
secondary research   92, 99–100
sensory analysis   95
sensory food properties   31–42
sensory testing   54–5
smell   36–7
snacking   64
social groups   60–1
spending patterns   62–3

spoilage organisms   78–9
starches   18–19, 24, 34–5
starchy foods   24
statutory regulations   72–3
sterilisation   84–5
stock rotation   83
storage of food   32–3, 44–5, 82–3
sugars   18–19, 34, 54
surveys   98
sweetness   54

T

take-aways   56
tamper-proof seals   87
target groups   97
task analysis   92–3
taste   36–7
teenagers   65
television programmes   99
temperature, spoilage   79
tenderising   55
texture   37
toddlers   65
trace elements   22–3
Trades Descriptions Act
    1968/72   72
traffic light labelling   88

U

unsaturated fatty acids   16–17

V

vacuum packaging   87
vegetable cooking   53
vegetable fats   16
vegetable protein   14–15
vegetarians   66
vitamins   20–1, 32

W

water   20–1, 28–9, 32
water soluble vitamins   20–1
websites   99
weight loss   67
Weight and Measures Act
    1985   72

Y

yeasts   78